Finding STRENGTH,
Finding LUMIES

J E N I F E R   H I G G I N S

ISBN 978-1-6384-4551-7 (paperback)
ISBN 978-1-6384-4552-4 (digital)

Christian Faith Publishing, Inc.
832 Park Avenue
Meadville, PA 16335
www.christianfaithpublishing.com

Printed in the United States of America

Thank you to my husband and my two beautiful children, Emie and Lucas, who have shown me what strength and determination are when life throws a curveball your way. To all the families who have experienced what it's like to have a child diagnosed with cancer, their fight, and the toll it takes on a family. It sucks, and it's hard! For those who have not experienced this, this book will show you, firsthand, my family's journey and that there is never a "normal" to go back to. There's only moving forward!

Chapter 1

THE DIAGNOSIS

"Your child has cancer."

September 9, 2015 started like any other day. During my hours at work, my son Lucas wasn't feeling well. He was prone to getting croup, so we thought that this was just another occurrence. Since I had to work, my mother-in-law was able to take our son into the doctor's office to get him checked. What we thought would be a normal doctor's visit with steroids and a possible nebulizer treatment turned into our worst nightmare. Our doctor's office at Kaiser was close to closing, and my son's primary care doctor thought our son didn't look healthy. She thought that he possibly could have a urinary tract infection, and since they weren't able to stay open past hours, she referred my mother-in-law to take our son to the children's hospital. She was able to take him to the children's hospital closest to us. My husband, Anthony, met her to tend to our son. I recall it was around 5:30 p.m., and this week of work happened to be my closing shift, so I would not be getting off until 6:30 p.m. Concerned but unaware of the actual health of my child, I chose to stay at work since I would soon be off. It was a debate of staying at work or leaving work and getting "an occurrence" for leaving work early. This is a whole other topic that will be discussed later! Since it did not seem that urgent, and I did not want to deal with the repercussion of leaving work early, I chose to finish out my shift.

After work, I headed up to a satellite portion of Children's Hospital in Broomfield. I work downtown, so this drive took me about forty-five minutes. Once I got to the hospital, I was escorted to the back where Lucas and Anthony were located in a room. I remember getting to the room, sitting down, and not even being in the room for about two minutes. In this short amount of time, Anthony filled me in that they were unsure of what was going on with our son and that they were running tests and waiting for results on his blood work. I feel that timing is impeccable! As soon as Anthony told me this, the doctor that was treating Lucas had walked into the room. I recall that she had this look of terror on her face, and she was hesitant to talk to us. We were sitting on the bed with Lucas on my lap. The doctor must have never had to deliver this type of news before because there was no filter or anything, and she just blurted out, "Your son has cancer. We don't have any answers, and we don't deal with this stuff, and his labs broke our lab machine because it's not designed for things like this, so we're transferring you to Children's Hospital's main campus located in Aurora." I can still remember that I felt like what she had said was unreal, and my brain to this day still is in disbelief at times.

All within about five minutes of being told that we would be transferred, there was an ambulance that had come for us to transport Lucas to the main hospital. Since he was only three at the time, the ambulance required us to get his car seat so they could attach this to the transportation bed that goes inside of the ambulance. I just stood there in shock. Thinking back to this day, I still don't know exactly what I did or how I felt. I feel that everything inside of me was just drained, and I didn't know what to do. I just recall going with the flow and doing as I was told. My husband, being a smoker, offered to go to the car to get the car seat. I think he partly did this because he knew I was not all there but also so he could smoke a cigarette and sink in what we were just told.

I can still recall the hospital, the hallway, the smell, and the sound of everything from this moment on. As Anthony came back with the car seat, I was holding Lucas in my arms. The EMTs put Lucas's car seat on the ambulance bed, attached it, and asked me to place him in it and buckle him in. I feel like everything from this moment was in slow motion. I was allowed to go in the ambulance with my son, and my husband had driven our car to the hospital to meet us once we arrived. I remember sitting in the ambulance with nothing crossing my mind besides thinking it was interesting that the ambulance was taking the toll road to get there the fastest. It was a silent ride, and I could tell that the EMT that was riding in the back was unsure of what to do. Finally, he broke down and asked what was wrong with my son. I just remember looking at him and quietly stating that we were just informed that our son had cancer. He had this shocked look on his face, and you could tell that he was unsure of what to say. All he could say was, "I'm sorry to hear that." Thinking back, we will now hear this phrase a lot throughout our journey. And when you're on this end of the spectrum, in all honesty, you just want to tell others to shove it because it means and does absolutely nothing for you. Unless a family has gone through this nightmare, you cannot even begin to imagine what goes on and how little these words mean. Trust me, I know. I've also been on the other end and have tried to empathize with others before this journey began. You try to be sympathetic, but no matter how hard you try, I've learned that it just becomes pointless. I did learn, however, instead of trying to say sorry or trying to feel a person's pain with the same experiences, it's easier and more meaningful to simply ask, "How are you doing?" Not only does this help with the person going through the treatment, but it also helps with their family members. A lot of times, we tend to forget about all the loved ones and forget that they are going through this traumatic event as well.

Riding in the ambulance, even with sirens on, felt like a lifetime. In actuality, I believe the ride was about forty-five minutes. Once we finally got to the main campus of Children's Hospital, we were taken to the emergency entrance. We were then taken to an ER room that was waiting for us. We sat in this room for about an hour before we were greeted by a doctor. Once the doctor had entered, our encounter seemed very brief. We were told that we were just waiting for a room to be set up for us up on the seventh floor, the oncology floor. Once we got to this floor, then we would be provided with more information.

Sitting in this room, Lucas thankfully was asleep at this point. After sitting for a few hours, I think it was around midnight when Anthony and I finally looked at each other in disbelief. Still, with no words, it was just a look of "is this happening?" We both finally broke our silence and said, "Is this happening?" In the meantime, we had to figure out other things as well. We also have a daughter who at the time was six. She ended up staying with my mother-in-law. I remember also getting multiple phone calls from my parents trying to receive information about what was going on. I finally caved, and the words came out of my mouth, "They said that Lucas has cancer." This shocked my parents as well. Our conversation, I feel, was brief as my mind didn't want to have to talk about the situation. All I can remember was my parents asking if we needed them to come up from Pueblo, which is a two-hour drive on a good day with no traffic. I had told them no as Anthony and I felt that we needed to figure out what was going on. Plus, we were still sitting in the ER room with no information to provide yet. We didn't even know what would occur from this moment on—talk about time standing still. Not realizing it, we sat in that ER room for probably four or five hours just waiting and waiting and waiting for a room to become available. The only reason that I can recall us sitting in this ER room with no movement was because of the last time I had talked to my parents. After I had told them not to come up until we had more information, here they were at our ER room. I think it was finally around 3:30 a.m. when we were told we were being moved because a room was now available for us up on the seventh floor, the oncology floor. We slowly took the elevator up and were taken to a room that was located in the corner of the floor on the northeast side of the building. This room, as we knew it, would become his room for a week, and, as we knew it, this hospital would become our second home.

Ironically, this next part seemed to happen so quickly, I'm not sure if I remember all that had happened. Not getting any sleep, the sunlight started to come up. Once the sun comes up, there is a lot more movement that occurs within the hospital. I think we had a doctor come in. I know we had some nurses, and, at one point, we had a social worker come in to talk to us. As best I can, I will try to recall this week to you in detail as I still sit here in shock and think back about all the crap my son had to endure. The doctors had come in and explained stuff to us, and, to this day, I don't remember what they had told us. I'm sure it was about what was going to happen and how they were going to treat our son. I do remember that Lucas was going to be assigned a doctor, a fellow, and a nurse. These team members would be specific to him and his treatment. They became like family who took very good care of Lucas. We couldn't have been blessed with better doctors and nurses to take care of our baby. We are forever grateful for them. From the first moment we met each one of them, I could tell Lucas was in good hands. This brought some relief, knowing you could trust those who are caring for him and knowing that everything that they do or will be doing is all in the best interest of Lucas and ensuring he is a cancer survivor.

Lucas was poked and prodded for the next week. When I mean poked, he had an IV that was inserted into his hand. Being a three-year-old stubborn boy and not knowing what was happening to him and why, he hated this. Lucas pulled out his IV several times that first day, which not only made it difficult to administer medication but also made it difficult to watch because they kept having to put in a new IV, which meant more poking. At one point, he had quite a few marks as they had to find a vein that they hadn't already used. Through his IV, he was given fluids and several medications. Watching your son be poked at and forced medication is not an easy process. Trying to help and comfort Lucas was hard. It was also a very difficult task trying to get him to take his medication. It was a difficult task in itself trying to figure out ways to give Lucas his medications as this was all new to us. We tried different flavors, such as chocolate and cherry syrup. Nothing stuck. Never have I been spit on so many times in my life. He refused to take any of the medications, and most of it wound up on me. From this day on, for three years, I will remember all the monitors and different hospital experiences. These experiences today, at times, still haunt me.

Early that morning, we finally heard from the doctors about Lucas's diagnosis and discussed what our plan would be to treat his condition. Lucas was diagnosed with acute lymphoblastic leukemia (ALL). We were also informed that the course of treatment to cure his cancer would take three years. We were provided with information about the treatment plan and what each cycle of chemotherapy would entail. At this time, we knew we would be in for a long haul of chemotherapy. But also at this moment, I didn't realize that his treatment plan was one of the longer courses of treatment for cancer. During this time, we were also given information about including Lucas in a study while he undergoes his chemotherapy regimen. We did end up agreeing to do the program as we learned that previous children who had participated are the reason that curing leukemia in children is more successful nowadays. My thought was that if someone is helping us so my child can be cancer-free, of course, I will make it to where we can help other children in the future. We also learned that there wouldn't be any additional requirements to do the study, extra specimens would just be taken during his course of treatment.

After a few hours of going into details of what would occur with Lucas and letting this all sink in, we were visited again by our social worker. She talked to us about resources and how they could help and how she could help if we needed anything. She also informed us that at this time, three years will seem like a long time, but in the end, we will see the light at the end of the tunnel. I could tell she was sincere and has had to talk to many families. She had a sort of comfort that I didn't know would put me a little bit more at ease. She also became someone I could rely upon over the years to help our family when it was needed. Even after treatment, she has still been here for not only my family but for me as a mother. I didn't know it at the time, but she helped me through in a way I can't explain. She taught me how to take care of myself so I could take care of my family. One of the things that still resonates with me from that day is something that she said. I will never forget it. She asked me what type of cancer Lucas was diagnosed with, ALL or AML. When I told her ALL, she looked directly at me and said with no hesitation, "Well at least your child has the better of the two types of cancer." At the time, I was thinking, *What is that supposed to mean? How is one type of cancer better than another? Cancer is cancer. It's all bad. I was just told my son has cancer, how on earth can you stand there and tell me that my child has the "better" cancer?* I'm pretty sure my eyebrows scrunched together, and I had this confused look on my face. During this time, we were also warned that things would get worse before they got better and that the next six to nine months would be our worst nightmare. These were the most horrifying moments of my life as a parent. Man, oh man, did they hit this on the nose! However, now looking back after it all, I understand it. It may sound odd, but it was nice to be given all the information upfront with no filters.

The only time that Lucas left his room during this first week was to go and receive an x-ray. This needed to be done to check his chest and muscles to place the port—talk about a long walk from one floor to another and back. I don't remember the whole journey, but I do remember a long, white hallway we had to walk down to get to the x-ray room. It was quiet, no one else was around, and it smelled clean. It also had windows that walked along the ground on the outside of the hospital. It must have been on the second floor because we were up higher than those that were outside enjoying the warm weather. The x-ray was difficult for Lucas as he was scared and didn't want to lay by himself. I had to place him down on an ice-cold bed and cover him with one of the hospital blankets so he wouldn't freeze. It took a couple of shots to get a good picture as he didn't want to lay still. But who could blame him?

This first week was rough. And although all of his treatment was rough, I can't say that this was the part that was the worst. In this first week, so much had occurred. Lucas was given his treatment plan, his first doses of chemotherapy, antibiotics, and was poked many times because they had to change out his IV line several times. At first we were not told how long we would stay. All we were told was that we would be staying until they could get Lucas's counts back to regular stability. So a week was what it took.

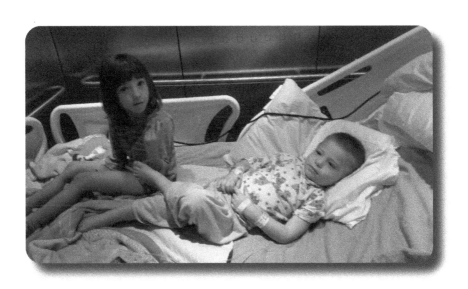

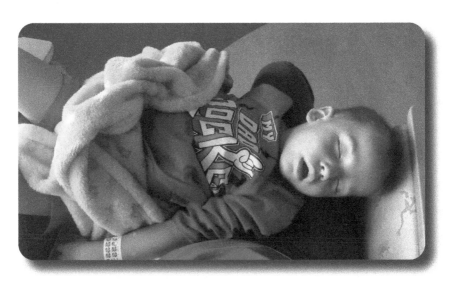

Chapter 2

THE NEXT STEPS

WHILE LUCAS WAS IN THE hospital, we were given the option to have a port put into his chest so he could receive his chemotherapy. This would be placed so he would not have to get an IV inserted into his arm to administer the medications he would be receiving. As with anything, undergoing surgery is always a big concern. This was nerve-racking as it would be attached close to his heart to allow the medication to be pumped through his main bloodstream. We did end up doing this, and his port was placed on September 11, 2015, just two days after diagnosis. We are glad that we chose this route. We didn't know it yet, but there would be many pokes for IV chemotherapy treatment.

The surgery took about an hour. For this, Lucas was transported from the seventh floor of the hospital down to the second floor where the surgery center was located. The waiting room was a small area with some couches, end tables, TVs, fish tanks, and another TV that gave updates on patients by their hospital record number. I remember sitting in the corner of the room where it was dark, so if I shed some tears, I would not be seen. I think for the entire hour it took for Lucas to go through surgery to get his port put in, my husband and I didn't speak a single word to each other. We just sat next to each other, both glazing out into the waiting area and observing other families that would come and go. During this procedure, Lucas also got his first bone marrow spinal tap done.

The port that Lucas received was a PowerPort. The easiest way of how I can explain that these devices work is the port is placed under the skin. Attached to the port is a catheter, which then is placed into the bloodstream so the medication can enter the blood. On the outside of the skin, there is a bump as to where the port is located. Each time the port needs to be accessed, we would put numbing cream onto it to minimize the pain. A long needle with a butterfly would then be placed into a certain spot within the port. Each time this would need to be accessed, this was the procedure that would occur. After the needle was placed, it would be covered with a bandage called Tegaderm to keep the butterfly in place and to cover the area so no germs could get into the blood. I do have to admit that this made it easier for Lucas to receive his treatments. At first it was hard to adjust to—to watch your child get poked with a needle and watch them cry—because they don't understand what is happening to them. However, over time Lucas became a pro. It's amazing how kids can adapt. His strength and inspiration got me through some dark days.

Before we could leave the hospital after that first week, we were required to attend a meeting that would provide us with some information on what to expect and what we would need to do as different situations would arise during treatment. This meeting, I feel, took about an hour. We went into one of the meeting rooms where we sat with three other families. It was awkward and difficult. We were asked to introduce ourselves and state what type of cancer our child had. Anthony is an antisocial person and does not like to talk in front of other people. So, of course, this fell on me to provide the information. I said my name was Jenifer, and my son was just diagnosed with ALL. I made it as brief as I could so I wouldn't have to talk long. I don't recall much of the other families and what they had talked about with their children. This was not intentional. I think it was just because my brain still wasn't understanding what we were doing at this hospital. I do remember a mom being there by herself and that her husband was back at home working. The only reason why I remember this was because she discussed that her son had a brain tumor, and they were flown on a Flight for Life helicopter from Wyoming—that and maybe because her son was diagnosed with a different form of cancer than the other two families that were in the group.

After the families introduced themselves, we were given a binder that had two sets of information with different tabs. They were titled the Family Handbook for Children with Cancer, and The Children's Oncology Group: Family Handbook. To be honest, both packets have the same information, but there are a couple of different tabs with different information. I'm still not sure as to why they just couldn't combine the two! They briefly discussed these and said that if we needed anything, there were resources in them that we could utilize.

We were also given a packet called "The Other Side of the Mountain: A parent's guide to surviving childhood cancer." Sitting here looking through all this information, to be truthful, I have not read a single word in this packet. I sit here just staring at it, wondering if I should have. But there's no point in dwelling on the past, and we got through our journey just fine without it. In a card pocket, we were given ten different business cards for ten different individuals who would be assigned to either Lucas or me. These included our social worker, child life specialist, financial counselors, physical therapist, and so on. You don't realize how many individuals it takes to take care of your sick child until it's placed right there in front of you.

Finally came the most important information: "A PowerPoint on Family Education." It was eighteen pages, front and back. This we would know like the back of our hands. The first thing listed was the important phone numbers. There was the twenty-four-hour, "on-call" number and Monday through Friday from 8:00 a.m. to 5:00 p.m. number. There were guidelines and when to call these numbers. We learned that something so little, such as a fever, is no longer considered a small concern.

We were taught what was required to call these numbers. We would need to call if Lucas had a fever, which is considered 101°F once or 100°–100.9°F two to three times within twenty-four hours, taken two hours apart. If a fever did occur, we could not give Lucas Tylenol or Advil as this could alter the readings of blood cultures that would need to be done. We also had to watch for shaking chills without a fever, earache, sore throat, headache, pain with peeing or pooping, pain not getting better with medicine, and redness, swelling, pus, or draining from anywhere amongst the body. All these could be a sign of an infection somewhere within the body.

Emergency room visits (ER) were next on the agenda. We would often feel like we were VIP every time we went in. When we showed up at an ER, we had to ensure that we wore masks, informed the security officer at the desk that we were bringing in a cancer patient, and that your child is *not* allowed to sit in the waiting area with other families or children. You could also call your doctor, which they would then call ahead to the ER to inform them that you were bringing in your child. This way they could be ready for us and could take us directly to an oncology ER room that was designated for cancer patients. We learned that there were two of these rooms. Each one we visited quite often. The only nice thing about being in one of these rooms was there was a bathroom in them, unlike other ER rooms where you had to go down the hall. I'm still not saying it was anything fancy as the toilet was placed behind a door, and then you would use a curtain to enclose the space. But it was nice not having to leave the room knowing your child isn't feeling well. You would also get drinks brought directly to your room as you are required to stay within the room for less exposure to germs.

Again, we were reminded that once you get to the ER, you need to ensure that you tell the staff your child has cancer. We were also informed that under *no* circumstances could they ever take our child's temperature rectally, give our child an enema or suppository to treat any symptoms. Once at the ER, if our child does have a fever, they will get blood cultures and start antibiotics within the first hour.

These were the most important factors that were addressed that day. Other things that we discussed were things that would happen during treatment, such as port placement, EMLA cream (numbing cream for the port), other uses for the EMLA cream (lumbar punctures, bone marrow aspirate), eating regulations for different procedures that would take place during the treatment when your child is put to sleep. We were told about the different cancer treatments specific to each type of cancer, chemotherapy and the side effects, the different types of blood counts on white and red blood cells, low platelet counts, blood or platelet transfusions, weight gain, weight loss, mouth sores, hair loss, and infection prevention. These are the only things that we discussed within the first twelve pages. The list continues, but we'll stop at these. I know, brain overload.

Germs—this word is something that we will learn a lot about, especially in such a small amount of time. I thought I knew quite a bit about germs, especially having a biology degree with a chemistry minor and having to learn about different bacteria in school. But, boy, was I wrong. There were so many things that we had to redo and relearn to make sure things were safe for Lucas. We could no longer share drinks, share silverware, or share anything really as we needed to make sure Lucas would not get any of our germs in any kind of way. Hand sanitizer and masks would also become a regular regimen within our house. We had bottles of hand sanitizers all over the house. I'm talking by the front door, the back door, in the kitchen, in all the bedrooms— pretty much in every room of the house. This helped with some of the eliminating of washing hands so much. It also made it easier when family and friends would want to come over to visit.

When Lucas was first diagnosed, we also had a dog that the kid's grandma had bought for them. At this point, we had to give it back to grandma. It was difficult, but it was in the best interest because the puppy would pee and poop within the house while we were trying to potty train her. With Lucas being immunocompromised, we just could not risk it. We also got our carpets cleaned and our air ducts cleared out as well. We figured we might as well start fresh and clean everything. We just couldn't bear to take any chances.

Another thing that we had to get and discuss with the doctors on the last day of his hospital visit was medications. On the first floor of Children's Hospital, there is a Walgreens pharmacy. This is here specifically to dispense medications for patients before they could leave. I can't recall how many medications that I had to get, but I think it was around eight to ten. When I went back to the room, we had an intern pharmacist come in and discuss the medications with us. He gave information on what we were receiving, the side effects, and the importance of each medication. I know that not all parents feel like this, but I feel for me this was a pointless conversation. I don't want to sound ungrateful, and there were a couple of questions that did occur during the conversation; but when you are around medications, it's kind of a mute discussion. I don't want to go into much detail about this right now, but I will inform you about this in a later chapter.

Finally we went home. From this moment on, our lives would be changed forever. We were often told that we would adapt to our new normal before too long. That was true, it didn't take long. It also didn't take long for Lucas to start his chemotherapy and begin his journey through this ordeal. I learned a lot about my kids, myself, and my marriage. You don't know how strong you are until being strong is your only option.

Chapter 3

CHEMOTHERAPY

THERE WAS NO TIME WASTED from when we left the hospital to when we got home. The day after we got home from the hospital, Lucas started medication. For this day, I had to give him four different medications. Some of the medications given are to help offset the side effects of chemotherapy. This was still not an easy task to conquer, Lucas was at first difficult to give the medications to. I don't blame him though, some of the liquids smelled disgusting. There was one that was mint flavor, and I wouldn't want to take it. For the medications that didn't come in liquid and only came in pill form, I had to crush these down with a pill crusher and give them to him through a syringe. Most often than not, it was simply mixing with water as over time his taste buds became altered because of the chemo, and nothing tasted the same to him. But at first, it was difficult.

After only being home for a day, we had our first visit to the inpatient clinic where we met with his oncologist and his nurse. This first visit lasted all day. This consisted of doing a checkup and labs and going more in-depth upon his chemotherapy regimen. Each month we would be given a calendar from his nurse that would serve as a reminder of appointments, medications, and labs. They also made time to answer any questions that I had. Lucas started with one nurse at the beginning of his treatment, but she ended up transferring to another unit within the oncology department. This nurse was great, but I feel that things tend to happen for a reason. His new nurse that took over his care is amazing. Neither her nor his oncologist or fellow ever made me feel out of place so to speak. No question or concern was dumb, and they always went out of their ways to address my concern no matter how little it was. They knew that to me, all my worries were legit and meant something to me. I think, from experience, they also knew that it would put a parent a little bit more at ease. Not once during his chemotherapy did I ever feel worried that he wasn't getting the best care. This to me is a big deal as you are putting complete control of your child's health in their hands and ensuring they do everything to make sure he is cancer-free.

As I stated before, we were warned that the first six to nine months would be the most difficult to get through. Even being warned, I still didn't think we would go through everything that we did. I'll try to explain this as best I can. Each time Lucas gets his labs drawn, they test for various things. But the main four factors they look at are his ANC, his hemoglobin, platelet counts, and red and white blood cells. These numbers are important because they determine how susceptible he can become to being ill and if he would need a blood or platelet transfusion. First is the ANC. This stands for absolute neutrophil count. This is such a long word and still makes no sense to me. But I do know the importance of it. This count determines how strong our weak Lucas's immune system is. We were informed that anything under 500 is a concern and that his immune system is very compromised. In other words, he's more likely to get an infection or become sick. Anything over 500 is good, but they would prefer it to be over at least 550 if I remember correctly. The hemoglobin is how much oxygen is within the blood. If this becomes too low, then a blood transfusion would be needed. They also do this with the platelets, white, and red blood cells. They are determining factors to how the medications are working and how his body is responding.

Within the first month of treatment, Lucas continued his course of medications. He also started a thirty-day regimen of steroids called dexamethasone. We went to the clinic for checkups and labs eight times. During this duration, he received IV chemotherapy, had another spinal tap, and got his labs drawn. So far all his labs were looking good. During a seven-day course, at home, I would give chemo every day that needed to be taken specifically two hours before or after a meal, and *no* dairy. I found this easier to be done at night while he was sleeping. I also couldn't find it in my heart to tell him that he could not eat after a certain time, so I would set my alarm for two hours after he last ate so I could wake up and give it to him. Usually, this was around 11:00 p.m., and after a bit, I would no longer even need an alarm. I adapted to an internal clock to where I would just automatically wake up. I would give a second chemo tablet one day a week on the same day each week. On the weekends, I would give him antibiotics. And depending on the side effects, I could give him an additional three to five medications each day. Give or take on dosage changes throughout the week, I was responsible for giving medication to Lucas every day. After some time, both Lucas and I became a pro. There were times where he would be telling me that he needed his medication and would refer to them by colors! He knew what colors his medications were and which days he needed to take them.

Although everything was going well, of course, things hit a bump. Within the first month, Lucas happened to get another round of strider, a more severe case of croup. Like I said before, he was prone to getting croup quite a bit. This case, however, turned into the worst case he's ever had and gave us some great scare. In the Denver Metro area, there are several satellite Children's Hospitals. Closest to us is the Brighton branch, which is only about fifteen minutes from our house. Because of how severe it was and the difficulty of breathing that Lucas was having to catch his breath, we decided to take him to this location rather than the main campus in Aurora. We figured that he would receive some steroids like he always does and possibly a nebulizer treatment. Usually, they do this and then we wait for a few hours. And if his breathing is better, we are released. This time, this was not how it went down. Within about thirty minutes, they had given him two types of steroids and nine doses of epinephrine. This did absolutely nothing for him. They figured that since this was too severe of a case, and they could not help with his breathing, they would transfer him to the main campus. It was so urgent that Lucas took a helicopter ride on Flight for Life. On his trip, he was attached to an oxygen tank to help him breathe. Anthony and I were also not allowed to take the helicopter ride with him due to space. As he took off in the helicopter, we got in the car and drove to the main campus of Children's.

Once we got to the hospital, we thought we would be meeting Lucas up on the seventh floor. We were advised otherwise. Because they could not get his breathing under control, we were told that we would meet him up at the ICU. It hit us that this was bad. We had to wait about thirty minutes before we could go into the room with our son. They had to get him from the helicopter, get him situated into a room, and ensure that he was okay. When we did finally get to go back into the room, there was a sense of relief that he was there, and he was doing okay considering that since none of the other medications were working, and he was still struggling to breathe, the doctors brought in a respiratory therapist. It was concluded that they would bring in a breathing treatment called heliox. Once again, my mind was blown. Learning and experiencing something new in just a short month was difficult. This tank was one of those big oxygen tanks, but an added ingredient into it was helium, hence the name heliox. We were told that the helium helps the oxygen become lighter so it can travel easier within the lungs to get more oxygen into the body without Lucas having to work harder to breathe. Of course this was not an easy task. It had to be delivered through a mask. What three-year-olds want are plastic masks pushing air into their face attached to their face—none. I think after being so tired and exhausted from everything going on, he finally fell asleep. This made it so he could finally get the oxygen that he needed. They laid the mask next to his face close enough so that he could receive the oxygen and helium but not so close that it woke him up.

No matter how many times you have to sleep on a hospital couch, it is always uncomfortable. That night, neither my husband nor I had gotten any sleep. There was lots of tossing and turning and checking on Lucas to make sure he was breathing regularly. The next day, he was doing better. We still didn't get to go home; we were transferred up to the oncology floor for another night's stay. They gave him more steroids, hydrocortisone to ensure that his lungs weren't still inflamed. They also kept him there to make sure his labs were okay and that his ANC levels were over 500 so we didn't have to worry when we went

22

home. When we were discharged and able to go home, they gave us more hydrocortisone to give Lucas for the next four days. We tapered down off of this medication until he was done. Our visits to the hospital always felt short-lived. We were back in the clinic two days later for another round of labs, chemo, and a spinal tap. I'm glad that they always put him to sleep using propofol while they shoved a long needle into his lower back to remove fluid to test. Each time they did this, they would also give him an IV chemo into his spine.

I knew that ER visits and clinic visits would be a lot at the beginning, but it certainly takes a toll on you. A week after his last spinal tap, we were back in the clinic for yet another spinal tap, more labs, and his flu shot. Just when you think that you get some relief for even just a moment, a fever spikes up. This day was Halloween, October 31, 2015. Not even two months in, and we got to try out our twenty-four-hour emergency phone number. Lucas had a temperature of 102°F, therefore we called, and in a short period, we were on our way to the main campus of Children's Hospital. All I'm going to mention at this moment is I'm very grateful for my family, especially my younger brother. At this point, he lived with us so he was able to watch over my daughter. She was disappointed, but they went trick-or-treating together. They even took Lucas's bucket and got candy for him!

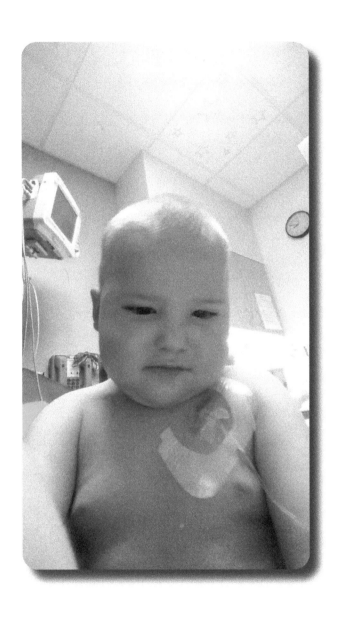

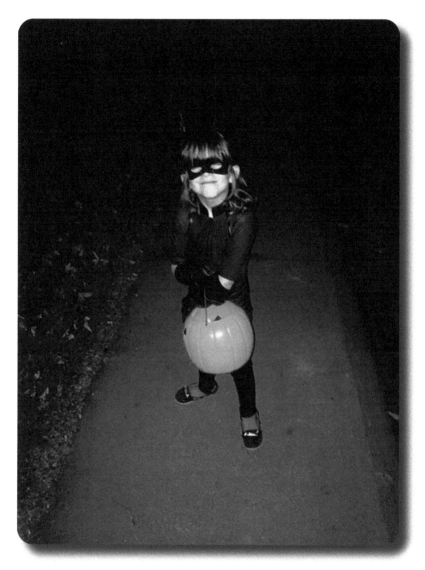

When we got to the hospital, I went and checked in with security, explained our situation, and told him that we were a call ahead. Anthony waited in the car with Lucas. Firsthand, how they treat cancer patients is very caring and very serious. Once they said they were ready for us, I informed Anthony. Once he got to the entrance with Lucas, we were given masks and greeted by a nurse to take us directly into the back. This was our first visit to one of those chemotherapy ER rooms.

Once we were in the room, we were greeted right away by a nurse. We were informed of what would happen. They checked his temperature, took labs, and started a culture. These cultures are put into a bottle that looks like a glass Coke bottle with some stuff at the bottom. They let this sit for an hour then do another set of labs for a second bottle. This one sits for twenty-four hours. After these two hours, since they have gathered his blood cultures, they give Lucas some Tylenol to help with the fever. We were there for about four hours before we were discharged and able to go home. Our daughter waited up for him so she could give him his bucket of candy. This was the very beginning of an unbreakable bond between brother and sister.

Two days later, we were back at the clinic to get yet another set of labs drawn. These were taken as a follow-up from his ER visit. They wanted to make sure that his labs were still good and that no other infection occurred in the passing day. Because of this and his temperature, we were put on precautionary measures. We were directed to go home and to self-isolate. This meant no visitors and that Anthony and I could not go to work for two days.

After all this, we were barely at the beginning of November. For the next three months, we managed to get by without any ER visits or croup. There were still seventeen visits to the clinic for chemotherapy, spinal taps, and checkups. At the beginning of December, Lucas also started physical therapy. He started to have some neuropathy in his legs due to a side effect of the chemo. It often made his legs numb. And while he was walking or running, he would often fall because he could not pick his legs up properly—talk about some scary moments watching your child be a child. As he tried to play and run around, he would often fall, and this was worrisome as a mother. Each time he would play, I would catch myself holding my breath, just hoping that he wouldn't fall. When you could tell he was going to fall, you just hoped that he didn't fall so hard that he would hurt himself.

In January, Lucas had to undergo an echo test so they could monitor his heart. This was to ensure that the chemo wasn't having any effect on his heart and that everything was going as planned. This testing took us about an hour. It was interesting to see all the different ways they use the sonogram to take pictures of his heart, the various ways that the heart beats and how they could measure his heart and lungs around it. For this visit, they gave Lucas an iPad and some headphones that he could watch as they knew this visit would take a while. They try to distract him as best they could as they had him move different ways around the table to capture different angles. I could tell this visit was a lot easier for him as he didn't have to worry about any needles. The only thing he had to worry about was the cold, gooey gel they use. Being ticklish, he often giggled throughout this visit.

Just when we thought we could stop and breathe and feel a sense of ease, things went south once again. Although this time, this time is where the nightmare begins. We were now in February, and we managed to almost get through this month without any complications. At this point, we were at a different point in treatment, which meant that we would be giving Lucas a new type of chemotherapy. They put a stint into his arm because for five days, we now had to administer injectable chemotherapy at home into his arm every night. This was very intense. The medication had to be refrigerated, which meant that when we gave it to him, it was cold. We would let it sit out for about five minutes to help reduce some of the cold, but we were instructed that we had to give it to him within this time frame. Anthony didn't like to have to hold our son in place and fight with him to sit so we could give him the medication. I would be the one who always felt like the bad guy. I had to get him on my lap, hold his legs within my legs, and hold his arms down tight so he would not move. Surprisingly, Anthony would be the one who would inject Lucas with the medication. Although he had a stent, and we knew where to put the medication, this process was still not easy. We had to be careful not to miss and poke him in his arm where he wasn't supposed to be poked. Anthony also did not like needles, so I feel giving the medication always took longer than it should have. Go figure! But after five days, we managed to get it done, and we were glad when it was over.

Of course, here we are again with croup. The same day that we finished this medication, Lucas had to go to the ER to be treated for croup. At least this time it was just a minor case, and our visit only seemed to last about three hours. What makes it interesting with croup is it always tends to pop up unexpectedly.

The next week, we decided to go to Pueblo to visit my parents. This was also a little bit of a break for us as my parents would help so Anthony and I could get a little bit of a rest. My mom would stay up to give Lucas his medication at night so I could go to bed and attempt to get some sleep. However while we were visiting, Lucas once again got croup. It never seemed to surprise me that we were always coming up with "solutions" to get through our day. Pueblo has *no* hospitals specific for children. And being a smaller town, there are only two hospitals to go to. We of course ended up going to the closest one. This episode took place around 11:00 p.m., so this would be a night of no sleep once again. When we got to the hospital, I went and checked in and explained our situation. This was challenging as the receptionist at the front desk didn't like what I was telling her. I also don't think they had dealt with many pediatric cancer patients, so they didn't have a protocol set in place like Children's Hospital does. Trying to explain to her that Lucas cannot be in the waiting room became exhausting. I finally just told her that when a room was available, then I would inform my husband to bring our son in. I also had to tell her multiple times that he had to be in a room that isn't around other patients—talk about an experience.

I sat in the waiting room for about forty minutes until we were finally told that we would be taken back. When we finally got to our "room," I think I had this thought of disgust because we were being stuck in a broom closet! I mean, I try not to judge, especially as I said before that they don't do many cases with kids with cancer. But I think they could have come up with something just a tad bit better. I can't say for sure, but I think that the reason that we had to wait so long was that they had to figure out where to put us to treat Lucas. This room was very small and only had two chairs that they must have brought in from the lobby or somewhere. It was not very clean. And in all honesty, it was a little creepy. Sensing that we would be here for a bit and not wanting Lucas to sit on one of these chairs, I placed him on my lap and cradled him to sleep while we waited.

After about another twenty minutes, a doctor finally came in. There was a tad sense of relief to know that he had dealt with cancer patients before and knew what we were talking about. He was concerned. And even though he was familiar with cancer, he wasn't an expert on the topic. I felt it very comforting the honesty that came from him and all the precautions that he took to make sure that Lucas was being treated for what he needed. Lucas ended up getting an x-ray, which was a different approach than we were used to. He shared the results with us and pointed out the inflammation on Lucas's throat as to where he was having difficulty breathing. Lucas was given a steroid to help with the inflammation. And once again, we saw a respiratory therapist. He gave Lucas a nebulizer treatment to also help. After this was done, the protocol is that we have to wait at least thirty minutes to ensure the medications are working before we can be discharged. I think it was finally around 4:00 a.m. that we were able to leave.

Due to Lucas's croup and getting it twice within a week, we decided to cut our visit for the weekend short and just go home. I guess this was a good call because starting Sunday, our lives would be turned upside down. Sunday, February 28, 2016, would be the day that would put things into a whole new perspective of life. Lucas woke up feeling fine, but sometime that evening, he ended up not looking nor feeling so well. I went to give him a bath, thinking this would help him feel better. When I took off his shirt to start to undress him so I could put him in the bath, I think I just froze and started to cry. His torso was covered in bruises. Not thinking of it at the moment because I was overwhelmed with panic, I called out to Anthony. I couldn't get any words out as I was crying, Anthony looked at me and said, "We need to get him to the hospital." We did as we always do, and we called the twenty-four-hour line and talked to the on-call doctor about what we saw. She told us that she would call ahead to the ER and that we had to get there right away. Again, at this time, I'm very thankful my brother had lived with us. It seemed to be a thing where I would just tell him, "We gotta go. You gotta watch Emie."

The same story as before, we got to the ER, checked in, and got taken to a room right away. They took his temperature and accessed his port. I don't recall if I've mentioned this before, but each time we have to take him into the clinic or to the ER for treatment, we always put on the EMLA cream and cover it with some Tegaderm. This way, by the time we get there, he is numb and doesn't feel the needle being placed in his port. This is "accessing" his port. Back to the visit. When we discussed what was going on and showed them Lucas's bruises, they turned their attention to both Anthony and me. I was not expecting it, and I understand that this is normal procedure for a hospital. But we ended up getting questioned by four different staff members to ensure that we were not abusing Lucas. As I said, I understand this is their normal procedure, but it felt like a huge slap in the face! *Here we are trying to figure out what's going on with Lucas and why he has all these bruises, and you're making sure that I'm not abusing my child?* I wanted to tell them some not very nice words at that moment in time. But I had to stop and remind myself that there are children who get abused, and they just need to make sure that Lucas is safe.

I don't even know how much time had passed by, but Lucas finally had his labs drawn, and cultures were started. I have to admit, when labs need to be done STAT, they are done very quickly. We received his lab results, I believe, within thirty minutes, if not sooner. Lucas's blood work showed that he was neutropenic. This meant that his white blood cell count was very low. To treat this and help get his counts back up requires a blood transfusion. Lucas was given not only a blood transfusion but also a platelet transfusion that night. They were able to stabilize Lucas's counts, but we were required to go to the clinic the next day for a follow-up visit.

Since Lucas was more prone to infections, we had to make sure that we wore a mask to eliminate germs, especially while walking through the hospital. Masks were normal for us as well, and surprisingly, Lucas didn't mind these. I think it was partly because we both sported them together but also in part because his mask had Mickey Mouse and Friends on his. March 1, 2016 was the following day that we went to the clinic for his follow-up. Because of his counts, we had to be in isolation, which meant that we went to a room that had a bed, TV, bathroom, and the essentials since we could not leave. Usually when we would go into the clinic, Lucas could roam the halls, go get some snacks or a drink, and wasn't regulated to his room. But this time, being in isolation, we had to stay put.

Over the past few days, even before this visit, Lucas also seemed to have a lot of diarrhea. Since he was in diapers, it was not pleasant to have to change these stinky things so often. This was different than you would normally have. It was runny, it was yellow, and it was very stinky. So of course, during our visit, I brought this up to his nurse. They ended up taking a sample of this to run tests on, and it came back that he had what was called C. diff. This is a type of infection that is found in the colon. So with Lucas having low counts and now having a bacterial infection, we would be admitted and would be staying on the oncology floor once again. I wasn't sure how long this stay would turn out. We were placed on the bone marrow transplant side of the floor, which meant that there were more precautions set in place. You had to wash your hands before you could enter; you had to be buzzed in; and because of his symptoms, if you wanted to visit, you needed to wear both a mask and a gown. Thankfully, since I'm around Lucas all the time, I wasn't required to wear the gown and mask.

Once we were taken to our room, we were provided the information about what would occur. Lucas would get IV treatment of antibiotics to help fight off the infection. If I remember correctly, he had to get the antibiotic three times a day for two weeks, which meant that we knew we would be there at least that long. During this time, Lucas also became swollen in his stomach and had a lot of pain. He was uncomfortable and seemed to cry a lot. It was very hard. No matter what I tried, I felt that I could never keep him comfortable. ·

Lucas was also receiving blood and platelet transfusion because his labs kept coming back unnormal. After two days, due to the pain and the transfusions, they did an ultrasound on his stomach. A technician came in and took pictures for about thirty minutes. This was sometime in the afternoon. During our wait for the results, Lucas still was not getting better. He kept going through both blood and platelet transfusions. During one of the platelet transfusions, he ended up having an allergic reaction. He woke up in the middle of the night screaming because he itched so bad and was covered in hives. They treated him with Benadryl, and it seemed to help, and it helped very quickly.

Each time they gave him a new transfusion, they would pretreat him and give him Benadryl first so he wouldn't encounter another reaction.

If you think it can't get worse, you are wrong. Since Lucas had really bad diarrhea from the C. diff, I was changing diapers a lot. He had gotten diaper rashes even before he was diagnosed with cancer. We would always treat it with Desitin and other creams or ointments prescribed by the doctor. However, this diaper rash did not want to go away. It had become so bad that it seemed to have burned off some of his skin on both of his butt cheeks, making it an open wound. We couldn't use wipes, because being an open sore, it burned, and he would scream. I hated changing his diapers because he was always in so much pain from this as well. We would use a squirt bottle and water to wash his butt off, but it became so bad and would not heal that the doctor had another doctor from the wound and burn unit come and take a look at it. I don't know what kind of cream it was, but we were given a cream they use on burn patients and some powder to coat his butt. This created a protectant layer, so each time he would poop, it wouldn't stick to his butt. It sounds gross and disgusting, especially since you wouldn't wipe it off each time. But it worked. It took about a week, but it finally got better.

Lucas was still having pain and discomfort throughout all of this. They treated this with pain medicine. I wasn't sure how I felt about giving my three-year-old pain medicine being so young and knowing that there is the risk of possible addiction. After a very long discussion with the doctor attending to him that day, we decided that it would be a short treatment, so we moved ahead. This did put him at comfort, which I was glad he didn't seem to be suffering from any of his pain.

Two days had passed, and that evening, we finally got his results from his ultrasound. I can recall sitting in a chair while Lucas sat on the bed, watching a movie. Anthony and my father-in-law were also in the room that night. As usual, they were talking about random stuff that guys talk about—hunting, fishing, cars, who knows what else. Then Lucas's fellow came in to check in on us and see how we were doing. I feel like whenever people ask this question, it's always a habit to just respond, "I'm good, and you?" Even if you're not good, you'll wonder, why didn't I just say, "I don't know," or "I'm feeling blah." Just say it like it is. Anyways, back to that night. After she had asked how I was, she then asked if we had been given the results from Lucas's ultrasound yet. I told her no, we were still waiting for someone to share the results with us. Well she would be the one to tell us. I could tell by the look on her face and her body language, she didn't want to be the one to tell us. But I guess she had to learn that since she was becoming a doctor, she would have to deliver bad news to her patients. Being our fellow, we had already known her for six months, so talking with her was very easy. She told me that the results showed that Lucas's liver was failing, he was suffering from VOD. This affects organs in the body and was being caused because of some of the chemotherapy we had given him. She explained this was why he was going through so many blood and platelet transfusions. His body was not functioning properly. At that moment, I just felt my whole body drained. She was still talking, but I had no clue what she had told me. I could also feel the stares of my father-in-law, Craig, looking at me. I don't know how I managed to, but I held back the tears as best I could. I could feel them building in my eyes, but there's something about not wanting to cry in front of other people. I'm pretty sure some eventually rolled down my cheeks. She kept talking, and after a minute, I came back to. I finally mustered up the courage to ask her what this meant and what we should do. To this day, I still don't recall everything she said to me. I do remember the important stuff: No treatment in the United States could cure this. We had two options, we could try different medications to see if they would reverse the damage, or we could do a trial of a "miracle drug" that could reverse the damage. It was a drug that was called Defibrotide, was not FDA approved yet in the US but would be within the next nine months to a year. After a long discussion about this and knowing how some of the medications work, we chose to do the trial of the Defibrotide. This would mean that we would be in the hospital longer because it could only be administered by the doctors, and it was an IV treatment. It was a twenty-one-day trial, so we knew our stay would be extended.

After the fellow left, I stood up out of the chair. I could tell that both Anthony and Craig were both looking at me, and Craig, I think, asked if I needed a breather. I don't remember what I said, but I think it either must have been yes, or I'll be back. I looked at Lucas, and my heart felt like it broke into a million pieces. I rushed out of the room and headed for the elevators. I would have taken the stairs as they are much faster as I was trying to get out of that place as fast as I could, but they only have stairs for emergencies. Trust me, I learned this the hard way when Lucas first got diagnosed. I went down a set of stairs and got locked in the stairwell for about twenty minutes because you needed a badge to scan to open the doors once you're in there! After I got outside, I walked to the end of the street. Around Children's Hospital, there are several sidewalks and trails as it is around another hospital and CU medical school.

I must have walked around for about twenty minutes just soaking in the air and crying until I had nothing left. There are no words that express what I'm feeling, how I'm feeling, or what to do. All I can do is pick myself up and keep going because my son needs me, and he needs me to be there to get him through this. So back to his room, I went. Once I got there, Craig left as I could tell he felt uncomfortable and didn't know what to say. Anthony and I may have talked, but I'm not certain. I'm the type of person that just bottles things up and just keeps moving along. He eventually went home as my daughter was at home waiting for him. Plus she was still in school, and he had to work the next day.

The next morning a doctor that is in charge of the trial came in and talked to us about it. We discussed what would happen if the medication didn't work. If it didn't, we could try a second round of the medication for another twenty-one days. If it still didn't work after a second time, he could be up for a transplant. I think I kept asking so many questions for what-ifs because that's where your brain goes that the doctor finally said, "How about we try the first round, see what happens, and then we can go from there?" After all of our discussion, we had to sign waivers and papers permitting for them to administer the drug and that this too could come with side effects and all the legal crap that goes along with anything nowadays.

That same day, March 4, 2016, he started the trial of Defibrotide. This would be day one of our stay. This visit was intense and long. Lucas was starting to feel better, and his counts were getting better.

But being accustomed to a hospital room and living there is rough. I tried to make it as comfortable as I could. I was brought a radio with a CD player so I could listen to music and a yoga mat. I was stocked up on groceries, those that didn't need refrigeration. The cabinets turned into my pantry. I used a portable DVD player to do workouts too. And I think Lucas and I had watched *The Avengers: Age of Ultron* at least one hundred times, if not more. During his naps, I was fortunate enough to be able to use a treadmill or a bike down the hall that was used for patients that needed to do physical therapy. Of course I had to make sure that it wasn't being used, and I always made sure to wipe it down well with wipes. Sometimes I would also go outside and walk around the hospital to get some fresh air and sunshine. It was nice to know that a nurse would peek in on Lucas while he was napping so I could try to have a little bit of time to myself.

Another factor that still sits with me was one of the times they had to change out Lucas's butterfly for his port. During this visit, we learned that they had to change out his port every seven days to eliminate the risk of infection. Therefore during this stay, Lucas's butterfly was changed out three times. Lucas was starting to become accustomed to having his port poked. We even had our routine of how to do this to make it most comfortable for him and less scary. He would sit on my lap, put his thumb in his mouth (he was a thumb-sucker), and watch a video on my phone. What made it difficult was since they were changing it out, they did not have time to put the EMLA cream on his port to numb it because they needed to cover it up again immediately. I knew that today would be the day they changed out his butterfly, but I was not given a specific time. My oldest brother happened to come up that day to visit Lucas for the first and only time during his course of treatment. While he hung out with Lucas, I went and ran on the treadmill down the hall. When I had about five minutes left on my run, I received a text message from my brother stating that there were nurses in the room to change out his butterfly. I responded that I would be there in a minute as I needed to wipe down the treadmill. It took me maybe two minutes to get back, and I walked into his room. I was mortified at what I had seen. Lucas was being pinned down on his bed while the nurses were already replacing his new butterfly—talk about a mama bear moment. I wanted to scream and cuss at these nurses and tell them this was unacceptable. To this day, this memory remains with me and upsets me. I know you shouldn't dwell on the past, but I wish that I would have had enough guts to say something to them. I don't like confrontation, so unspoken, I remained. I was furious inside. Thankfully, Lucas was young enough that he does not remember this moment.

The oncology floor also has a break room. I was able to store food in it, and thankfully, they have a Keurig machine with coffee that I could utilize every morning! Our morning routine after we got up consisted of me going to get a cup of coffee and Lucas a cup of hot chocolate! The break room also had a freezer full of ice pop popsicles. I don't know how many trips I made a day to get a popsicle for Lucas. He loved these, and they seemed to make him happy especially since he was not able to leave his room.

The rules on this floor were intense, and I understand why. The prevention of germs was key. Each time you left a room and entered a room, you were required to use hand sanitizer. I used a squirt of sanitizer probably at least fifty times a day. Now this might be exaggerating somewhat, but it was a lot. Each time you went to the break room and came back, you would use it at least four times going in and out. You had to make sure that you wiped everything down behind you, especially in the break room. There was another small room designated for water and ice. You could only use their cups and lids and straws to get the water. If you put food in the refrigerators, you had to use a label and a sharpie to put your name and the date on it when you placed it in the fridge. I don't remember the exact time frame, but I think it could only be left in the fridge for maybe seven days. This may even be pushing it. After this time, it would be thrown out. If you did not put a date on it, it would be thrown out. It was a lot. But after a few days, you become used to it.

This was our life for the next twenty-one days, a total of twenty-four if you count starting from the day he was first hospitalized. Each day Lucas had a checklist of three items he had to check off. Bath, brushing teeth, and changing the sheets to his bed. Of course Lucas didn't change the sheets. It was either me or one of his nurses who did it. They always offered. I think it was part of their job. But I always felt guilty having them do it. Each time you changed the sheets, you also had to wipe down the plastic on the thin mattress of his bed and all the railings of the bed. Trust me, they ensure you are not getting any germs. I also had to change the sheets on my bed as well. You can't call it a bed, but it's where I slept. It was the couch next to the window that pulls out into a small bed. They brought me two pads to lay on so it wasn't so hard. It didn't help much, but at least it was something.

This stay made it difficult for visitors and especially hard on Emie. Anytime someone came to visit, we were only allowed two people at a time. They had to put on a gown and mask to come into the room. The visitors that we did have didn't seem to mind. Although I guess if they wanted to see Lucas, they didn't have the option to mind nor complain. The hardest part was with Emie. Because this was during flu season, the hospital was on lockdown, and no one under the age of thirteen, I believe, could go and visit. This meant that Emie and Lucas didn't see each other for twenty-four days. It was hard. It was hard not only on me, but it was also hard on Anthony. He was responsible for Emie at home this entire time. He had to feed her, bathe her, take her to school, get her ready for school, and all the other things that go along with kids. This was hard for him. And thinking back, I have to laugh. She always made it to school, but I think he always had a hard time with her hair. It was so thin and frizzy, it was hard to do, and he could never get it right. I even remember the first day after we got out, and I went to pick her up from school. Her teacher told me she could tell I was home because Emie's hair looked good that day!

It took about a week for the C. diff infection to get better. His antibiotic treatment for this was two weeks total. Lucas's diaper rash finally went away after about two weeks as well. And on day 21 of the trial, we were finally given good news. Lucas was back to being healthy, and we were able to go home. This was March 24, 2016, the longest and most grueling days of my life. But we felt like we were finally free. Lucas couldn't wait to go outside and feel the sun for the first time in a while.

As I said, that day, we went and picked Emie up from school. It was a surprise to her, and she was ecstatic. She and Lucas sat there and hugged for probably two minutes. When we got home, they went into the backyard and played on their playground for the entire afternoon. My birthday was also three days later, so it was a nice present to still have Lucas with us and to be at home.

After this, things started to finally look up. There were no ER visits or croup incidents. We had in-clinic visits for chemo and PT visits as well. May 24, 2016 finally arrived, and this was the day that he would start maintenance chemotherapy. Lucas was in remission and now doing treatment to keep cancer from returning. I would still be giving him his medications at home, and he would still need to go to the clinic for labs and checkups, but the frequency would now taper down to fewer visits. As time went on, our regimen changed. There were some hiccups due to dosage changes and his ANC dropping too low, so a few times, we couldn't change the dose of his medications. But this was minor and normal, considering everything we had already been through.

Of course the week before chemotherapy would end, we had to go out with a bang! Lucas wasn't feeling well, and we ended up staying in the hospital for a week for croup and a fever while he recovered. This visit consisted of antibiotics and medicine to help treat the coup. Since we knew that we were close, it made things a little easier. But of course there are still always worries and if this could affect his end date of chemotherapy.

Finally, November 20, 2018 arrived. It felt like forever to get to this point, but we had made it. It was a little stressful and nerve-racking as I would be stopping all of his medications this day, and our next visit with the doctor wasn't until the following week. When we did finally go into the clinic, this day was special! We were done chemotherapy, and we would finally be informed of the next steps. Three long years, and we were done! Lucas was given a cake to celebrate his end of chemotherapy day. The hospital also has a bell on their floor that all kids get to ring as a celebration of finishing. Lucas rang this bell for probably five minutes. He was given an award stating he finished his chemotherapy, and we celebrated with his doctors and his nurse.

This visit also came with a sense of relief and fear at the same time. We were once again given information. This time it was information on how to live life after cancer. It was strange, and I wasn't quite sure how I felt. There was some nervousness as you always worry about the possibility of cancer returning as well as all the things that could occur in the future as side effects due to the treatment he went through. But we can't dwell on any of that. We can just live life one day at a time and cherish everything that we have and truly be thankful for it. This was the first time the entire family had gone to an appointment. It was Anthony, Emie, Lucas, and me. I took many pictures and videos to cherish the moment.

After this, a lot of people kept telling us, "Oh, now you can go back to normal!" Normal, what is normal? What does that mean? The last three years have been normal for us. This was what we had become accustomed to. It isn't going back to normal because you can never go back to things like they were before. So once again, we needed to find our new normal.

Besides this, we would still be visiting the clinic. Over time it would decrease with the number of visits. But regardless, Lucas will be tested for the rest of his life to ensure that the cancer hasn't returned.

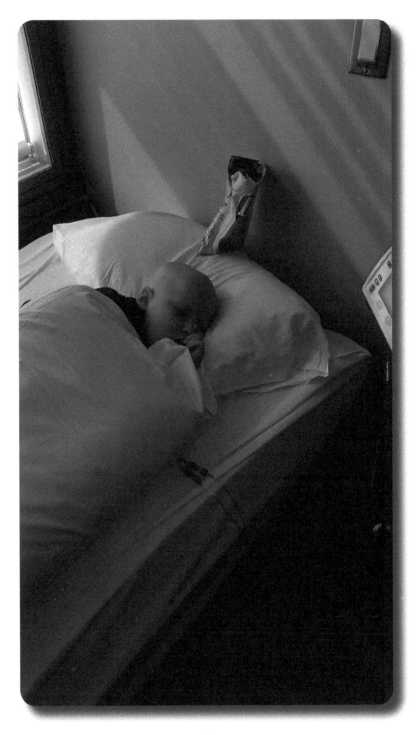

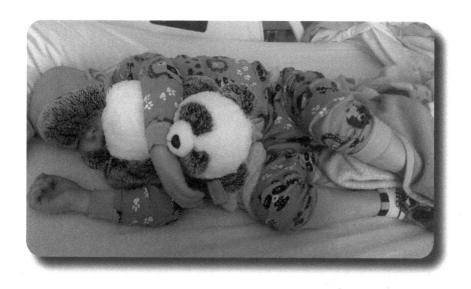

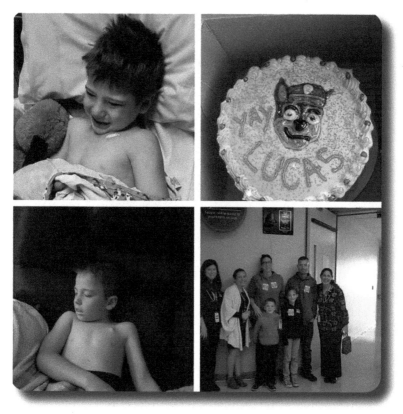

Chapter 4

SIDE EFFECTS

BALD—THAT IS THE NUMBER ONE thing that comes to mind when people think of cancer. It certainly was for me when Lucas was first diagnosed. But along with becoming bald also came chubbiness, skinniness, roid rage, and weird cravings. Within the first couple of weeks, Lucas lost his hair. It was a sad and shocking moment as to how this happens. I thought it would all just fall out at once. It didn't, it fell out in chunks. It started as one big patch in the back of his head. Then a little bit later in the day, another chunk on the side fell out. At this point, he had patches of hair missing from his head. It was sad to watch him start to lose his hair. When we would cuddle, I would always run my fingers through his hair as it was soft and thick and beautiful hair for a boy! Now I wouldn't be able to do this anymore.

We knew that all his hair would eventually fall out. But instead of just letting it fall out, Anthony took his hair cutters and buzzed his hair off. By the end of September, Lucas was completely bald. It took about a week for him to fully lose all of his hair. He was such a handsome little baldy, and he sported it so well. I also think that being young didn't allow him to know about being self-cautious. The baldness is also different in the fact that his entire head was smooth and shiny. It's not like men who go bald but still have some hair in spots and just cut it short. Since I was no longer able to play with his hair so to speak, I became fond of rubbing his little soft head!

Within the first month of treatment, he was also on steroids for thirty days as I mentioned before. Steroids are not fun, and they change your body in many ways. Lucas gained weight. I think at one point, for only being three, he weighed around forty pounds. He became bloated, didn't have much energy, and always seemed to be tired. He was always so energetic and active, that this was a different pace for him. He had a hard time going up and down the stairs to get to his bedroom. Many times he was too tired to go anywhere, so he found his best napping spot on the first step of the staircase. Surprisingly enough, he didn't seem to get cold. He always ran around and slept in a diaper.

One day—thinking back, it's a little bit funny now and sincerely cute, but at the time, it was heartbreaking—he tried to get on the couch to lay down and failed. He failed miserably. He tried backing up and running up to the couch to get up, but he failed several times. Being a stubborn boy, he did not want my help. It was like watching in slow motion. He couldn't move very fast, so his run was slow. And by the time he took the four steps to get to the couch, he couldn't get up. His stomach would hit the cushion, and his legs would dangle as he tried so hard to pull himself up onto the couch. After several attempts, he gave up and asked for my help. I was also selfishly glad because this meant that I got to cuddle with him.

When we went places, we got a lot of stares. They stared at him because he was bald and overweight. This always made me feel uncomfortable. It made me wonder what they were thinking. But after a while, I learned to not care. My son is going through something that has to be ten times harder than most people who experience difficulties in their lives. While you're in public, and you're buying your kid a candy bar and a bag of chips, you sure do get a lot of stares from strangers, not good stares either.

The reason that Lucas gained weight was because of the steroids. He was on steroids for a month straight. We were told that this was to help get his body get ready for the chemotherapy, and this was part of the regimen. Steroids are not fun. And when people talk about roid rage, they are not joking. He would become angry, hungry, and irritated all at the same time. Trying to deal with a three-year-old who doesn't understand what is happening to him and give him what he wants is maddening. Not only would he get angry and often throw things or just scream, but you also could not feed him fast enough.

When you are on steroids, you have an increased appetite and become hungry all the time. Or so at least with Lucas, it sure felt this way! He became so impatient when he was hungry that he learned how to use the microwave. No joke, what child at three years old not only learns how to use the microwave but wants to use it? I mean, it's not like he went all out and would make extravagant meals. I'm talking, he would warm up frozen waffles and know what button to push to make it warm. But still I have to give him credit. He was very determined to feed himself when he got hungry!

Throughout treatment, I feel like rules don't apply to your child. They go through so many changes with so many side effects that you have to constantly tend to what they need at that specific moment in time. So Lucas did not have a "healthy" diet. He often craved chips. Any kind of chips became his go-to—I feel like that and a McDonald's Happy Meal. I think at one point in time, we should have invested in a stock with McDonald's because all he wanted to eat were french fries. Salt, it seemed—like chips and fries—were his favorites. But anything with salt is what he craved! Now before you judge, don't worry, we checked with the doctors on what we were feeding our son. This was normal. Because of the chemo, taste buds often change, and sometimes things have no flavors or just no longer taste good. So don't worry, we were doing things right. I always made sure that we were.

It took about three months for Lucas to lose weight. Looking back at pictures, it was about mid-December 2015 when Lucas started to get back to his weight before being diagnosed with Leukemia. After this came the skinniness. He was still bald, and I think he started to get his hair back at the end of December. This took about a year for him to fully get his soft, luscious little blond locks back. And I was excited! Don't get me wrong, I loved him either way, and it's one of those catch-22 things. I had gotten used to the bald and his soft head, and now the hair felt weird. Lucas stayed skinny for a few months and then balanced back out and maintained a healthy weight throughout his treatment.

One thing that I was always thankful for was that he didn't experience any nausea or vomiting or constipation that came with taking these medications. In the beginning, we gave him medications to help with these; but after a few months in, they were not needed. I feel that he is so strong and resilient that he often inspired me to keep going forward. I was also thankful that we didn't have to go through this, because from those children we saw at the hospital who did experience these side effects, it seemed even rougher. I think that throughout this whole journey, Lucas was the "unnormal" kid going through cancer. He didn't have nausea, vomiting, constipation, or chills. He always kept going even when he didn't have much energy. I'm talking that it was so unusual that instead of him having chills that most people experience, he was a little heater. He would often sweat at night.

I briefly discussed this before, but Lucas did experience neuropathy in his legs. To help treat this, he did physical therapy (PT) at least once a month for quite some time. He also was sized and given shoe inserts to help when he walked. He liked his therapist. She was nice and always ensured he would participate even when he didn't want to. Lucas is a shy boy, and going with others is hard for him. So I often participated as well. We would make a competition out of it to see who could do it better. Of course he always beat me!

Lucas often felt pain in his hips as well. It wasn't extreme, but I think it was one of those pains that were always there, always constant, and over time becomes kind of miserable. Over time, this also went away as the PT helped with this too. The exercises that he did helped with his muscles and to make sure that his movement stayed on track. I think it was once Lucas got to his maintenance chemotherapy, we didn't attend PT anymore. His body was starting to shift, and the medications became a regimen that his body had gotten used to over some time.

Now I'm sure there could be other side effects that he had encountered, but these are the ones that stand out the most and the ones that were the biggest factors during his treatment.

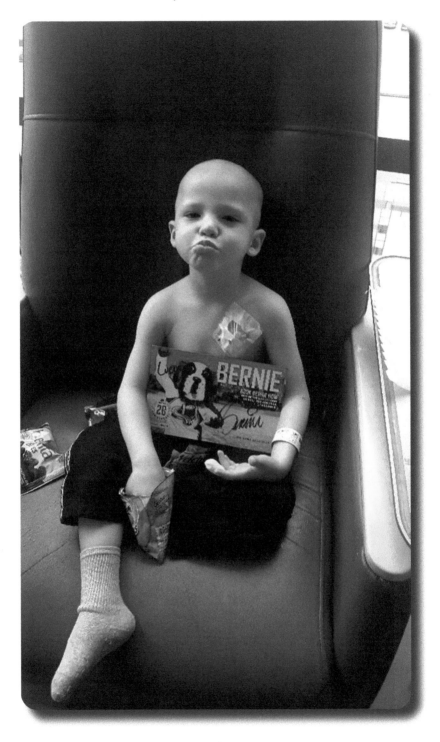

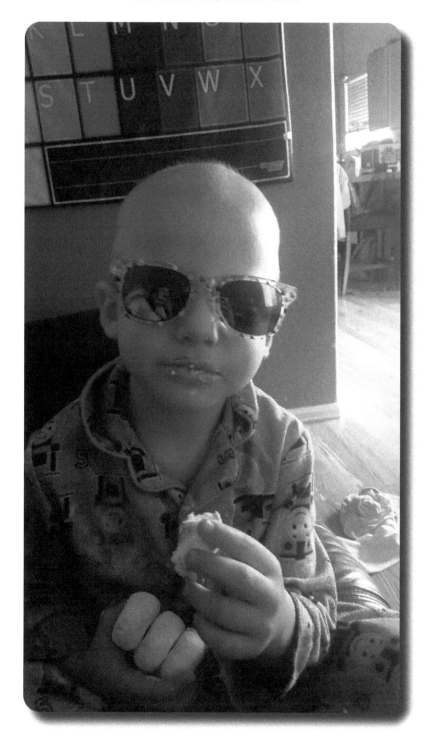

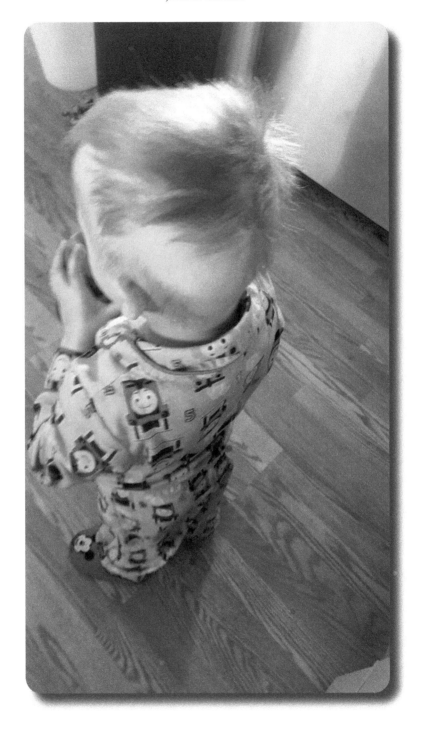

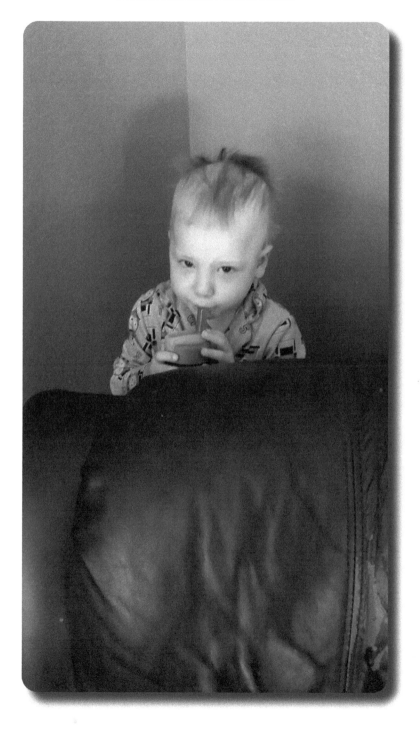

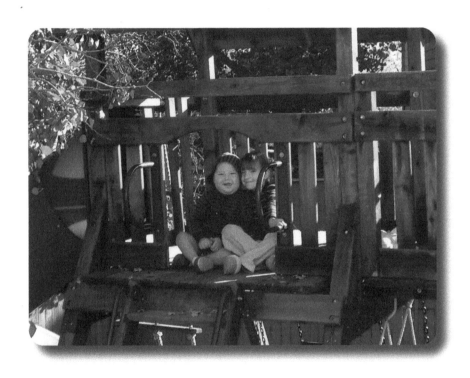

Chapter 5

SUPPORT

It's amazing the different support you receive from not only friends and family but from nonprofits as well. Working for a health care company, I have to admit that I have great health insurance. It is a plan that over time, I learned, covered a lot of Lucas's medical expenses. With that being said, don't get me wrong, the bills still racked up. For as many times as you are seen in the clinic, medications, the ER visits, the ambulance ride, the helicopter ride, and all the other things that come up along the way add up over time. I was working fewer hours due to making sure Lucas always got the care he needed. This decreased the hours I worked. I quickly ran through my vacation and sick time in no time. Thankfully, my company has a program that allows other employees to donate up to a week's worth of their vacation times to other employees under the circumstances that it is used for FMLA reasons. Of course I qualified for this. Having a brother who also works for the company is a benefit. Not only did he donate me hours, but he also got other employees within his department to donate hours to me as well. Along with this was an amazing pharmacist that I work with. She put up signs asking the staff that I work with to donate. I didn't expect it, but she truly worked her butt off. She asked every employee that came through the pharmacy to donate hours even if it would only cover a few hours. Between my brother and her, I think I ended up getting enough donated hours to cover about a month and a half of the time for me to be off. Of course this was all dispersed and used during the long hospital visit and a few weeks after so we could adjust when we got back home from our stay. This helped somewhat at the time, as I stated hospital bills started to roll in.

Shortly after Lucas got diagnosed, my sister-in-law (I call her this even though she's not "technically" married to my brother-in-law because we have a great relationship, and I've known her for as long as I've been married now) started a GoFundMe account for Lucas. Through this, she was able to get money donated to us from friends, family, and those that chose to donate anonymously. This helped pay some of the bills and keep us afloat as best that we could.

Through a coworker and our social worker, I learned about different nonprofit organizations. I feel bad for saying this, but some helped us tremendously that I do not recall their names. I also think that this was because the social workers would have us fill out an application, and they would submit so we weren't always sure where support was coming from. We were fortunate enough to have these organizations pay our mortgage and our gas bill for two months. The thought that there were organizations out there and people who donate to help fund families in this way always made me cry. Often at times, I felt kind of awkward asking for help, but I was always kindly reminded that these are why these programs exist. I cried a lot during these times because the help was very appreciated, and it ensured that my family was looked out for while we focused on Lucas's health.

Each month, the American Cancer Society would send us funds that would cover enough gas to get to and from the hospital for our appointments. This helped us out a lot since, at the beginning of treatment, we were going a lot. There With Care was recommended to me by a coworker. I don't even know where to begin with for this nonprofit. They provided various services to our family, things that I could never have imagined. They would send us some groceries every week so we always had food. They would send in a cleaning service once a month to clean our house with the essentials. They would send us a prepaid gas card to use at gas stations for gas. They would send both the kids care packages, activities to do. They sent us diapers, wipes, cleaning supplies, clothes, and, I mean, I feel the list goes on and on. They truly seemed to have thought of everything. I mean, when you're going through something like this, who even thinks about groceries or cleaning your house? I have to admit, it took a lot of stress off me to know that I didn't have to think of the everyday things and worrying about getting them done on top of what I was dealing with. It was amazing. And the employee who always talked with me to make sure we had everything we needed was awesome. Christmas that year was also covered because of There With Care. They had donors "adopt" our family to provide gifts. I just expected a few gifts for the kids, but they even gave something to my husband and me.

Shining Stars is another organization that we were lucky enough to come across. Although the kids still aren't old enough yet to participate in some of their activities, they were also there for us in other ways. We were invited to their annual Christmas party. I was just expecting to go and have lunch. Wow, they know how to treat kids and throw parties. They gave raffle tickets to the kids so they could put their tickets into a jar to try to win one of many prizes. Santa also visited, which was exciting for the kids. Then they had three rounds of picks that each child got to go pick a gift out amongst many tables full of gifts to take home. Both kids came home with new toys. And Lucas, that year, came home with a brand-new bike that he won in one of the raffles. He was excited and couldn't wait to ride his new red bike. Unfortunately, it was a little bit too small for him, but he managed for as long as he could.

There's the Ronald McDonald house. They made it so my parents could stay there for a few days at a time and come to the hospital to help out.

I am probably going to forget some people, but I do want to acknowledge and thank all of those individuals and foundations that had helped us get through this. It truly has meant a lot. You learn a lot about people and realize that there are still many great people in this world. This was also very helpful for us as we did not qualify for any assistance through our government. We tried to apply for Medicaid. We were denied because we made too much money. We could, however, pay to have Medicaid. This blew my mind. It's like, what on earth makes you think that I can afford to pay for my son to have Medicaid as secondary insurance with everything going on?

We tried to receive money from social security. This was also a no-go. Lucas was considered to have a disability even though it would be temporary. Once again, we made too much money. I think the only way we could have qualified for any assistance was for me to quit my job. Of course I couldn't do that. I'm the one who holds our insurance, and we need this to cover Lucas during treatment. It still baffles me that this is how things work. You have a working parent who still goes to work to provide for their family and ensure that you keep your insurance, but your government won't help you, and the only way they will is if you quit your job and make less money. It makes no sense to me at all. During all this, even with the medical bills and the struggles, we made too much money for anything. We didn't even qualify for reduced lunches or free lunches for my daughter at school. Trust me, this small bill was not so small, and we struggled to even pay this. Once again, I am thankful for all the outside help that we received.

One cool thing that we did get, as my brother bought it for Lucas, was a playhouse to put into our backyard. Since Lucas couldn't go anywhere and couldn't be exposed to germs, we were now putting one up for him. There have been so many people that have helped us throughout this, it is hard to even say thank you as these words don't seem enough. I had an uncle send us $1,000 to use toward the bills. At one point, we even received an anonymous letter in the mail. After I opened it and read the letter and saw what it was, I bawled. I think I bawled for probably about five minutes if not longer. It was a letter with advice and support, and included were two money orders totaling $1,000. To this day, I'm still in disbelief that we came across someone so caring.

My parents helped when they could. They would help us with groceries or gas and even helped us pay for Emie's school lunches. One of the biggest ways that they helped was also to help watch our kids. Even though it was hard, at times for a few days during the summer, the kids would go and stay with them. This is a big task as not only do you worry, but you have to trust that whoever is caring for him would make sure to give him medications as well. I have wonderful parents, and my mom beforehand even learned his regimen of medications that needed to be given at what time and on what days. This also took off some stress having to worry about babysitting, paying for a babysitter, and taking more time off from work. I won't lie, it was not easy as being the type of person I am, I don't like to ask for help, and I always wanted to make sure that everything was correct. Over time, I learned to accept the help, and I'm glad that I did. There were also weekends that my parents would come up and stay at the hospital overnight when Lucas was in for his long stay. This made it, so I was able to leave and go home, shower, try to have a break, and spend time with Emie.

To my coworkers and my work mom, big shout out. While I was in the hospital, they put together a care package for me! It included stuff from people that wanted to help out in other ways. I got a coffee mug, some candies, a new workout outfit, and oh geesh, so many other things that I am drawing a blank on. Sorry, y'all! I also got a Dazbog gift card from a coworker to use at the kiosk in the lobby of the hospital. I had a coworker come to the hospital to check in on me as well. She brought me some amazing food and Lucas a basketball hoop to play with in his room.

The biggest support of course was my family. My brothers and sister-in-law were tremendously helpful. They checked in a lot to see how I was holding up. At times I felt spoiled. One of my brothers worked close to the hospital, so he would often visit us in the hospital for lunch. He would bring me drinks, food, everyday essentials I may need, and most importantly support. He would also bring items to spoil Lucas and gifts from his daughters. One time he even brought Lucas new pajamas and a few other clothes that he could hang out in. Lucas ended up collecting a lot of toys during his stay from various people. Even my sister-in-law's parents showed support. They sent Lucas some toys, a wooden train set to play with. And they sent snacks for me as well. I'm a huge water drinker, so I ended up with a lot of flavored waters to drink! It was all very thoughtful, even just the small stuff. They also contributed a lot to my cabinet pantry!

So many people were involved in helping us throughout our journey, I feel that I may be missing some of you. If I am, it's not intentional. Truly, to all of those out there who were a part of our journey and contributed help in any way, we are very, very thankful for every one of you.

Chapter 6

WORK

I'll start with Anthony's work. He works for an electrical company. And throughout this whole ordeal, his company was amazing. Never once did they question any time he needed to take or penalize him for needing to have a day or take time off to help take care of Lucas. Heck, I don't even think they ever made him fill out papers for FMLA to protect his job. I guess this is the perks of working for a family-owned company. The lady that works in the office and does the HR work always went above and beyond to provide him with information and was great at checking in with him to make sure he was okay. She never seemed to question anything he needed. To this day, she'll still check in with him to see how he's doing and how Lucas is doing.

Not only did they never punish my husband for not being at work, but they also made sure that Lucas was doing good as well. The first week that he was in the hospital, his company sent Lucas a big box filled with goodies. It was filled with some movies, a portable DVD player, crayons, markers, coloring books, stuffed animals, and plenty of new toys. It even included a gift card for us to buy groceries. At the time, I don't think he could have worked for a better company.

The company I work for, on the other hand, showed no support for me whatsoever. I guess this is the reality of working for a big organization. Even though I work for an insurance company, I have to admit that the only two reasons that I am still at this organization are because you cannot beat the pay for being a pharmacy technician and the benefits. And of course, as you know, the benefits are a huge factor. Don't get me wrong, I fully understand policy and procedure. Heck, for the past ten years, I've been following them. But unfortunately, after going through something that I have gone through, you realize that the big companies show absolutely no appreciation for their employees.

Once Lucas was diagnosed and after we had gotten out of the hospital that first week, I had to also figure out my situation with work. I had FMLA papers filled out so I would be covered for taking the days off I needed to get Lucas to his appointments and whatever else would come up. What I had to learn—and learn the hard way—was that FMLA comes with stipulations, just like anything else. Yes, FMLA protects you and your job while you are out for various reasons. But what I didn't know was that with FMLA, you only get to take 365 hours per rolling calendar year. What this means, in my case, was that Lucas's FMLA started in September, so within the next year, I could only use 365 hours during this entire duration. You would get hours back as time rolled around again. Well, I bet you can't guess, and if you did, you guessed it right. I ran out of hours within the first five months of his treatment. So what this meant was now that if I took any additional time off, I was at risk of losing my job. I tried to talk to anyone and everyone that I could about my situation. Nobody seemed to care. At this point, we were going through a manager change, so I was dealing with upper management filling in within the pharmacy and taking care of our staff. As I said, I understand rules and policies and why they are set in place. But I feel like for certain circumstances that come up in life that are out of your control, there should be some exceptions. After talking with one of the team members in charge, I was told that there was nothing that they could do to help me. I was already able to take a part-time position going from working forty hours per week to working thirty-two hours a week so I could have one additional day off during the week to help eliminate some of my time off. This was helpful but not in a way that could tremendously help me at this point. After talking with several managerial staff members, I was finally told that there was nothing they could do for me. My options were either to continue working—and again I'm still showing up to work as much as I can—and risk my job. Since my FMLA was going to be exceeded, it could no longer protect my job. And this meant that according to company policies, I would be put on different levels of action for being gone. After so many additional days of being gone, you get through what they consider five levels. When you hit this point, you have a day of decision. You have to write a letter stating why you should still have your job. Even if you get to keep your job at this point, the next time or two, you are gone; you'll still be fire. So this route felt extremely pointless. The second option is to take a leave of absence from work. Of course this didn't feel like a very good option as I would be going unpaid. After you take a leave of absence, and you go unpaid for thirty days, you lose your benefits. I felt like I was being placed in a crappy situation. I honestly couldn't believe that a company that you commit to working for is not willing to do anything to help you in unprecedented times.

After struggling with this for a week, unsure what to do, I guess—as the phrase goes—"time is of the essence." In my case—I hate to look at it this way—eventually it all worked out. After struggling with what to do for the week, this was when Lucas was hospitalized for his lengthy stay when his liver started to fail. Like I said, crappy. But at this point, I guess my company got what they wanted. I would take a leave of absence from work. This was also where my coworker came in and got me enough donated hours to be able to get paid during his stay. This not only allowed me to still get paid, but it also allowed me to keep the benefits that I needed.

After this incident, I lost all respect for the company that I work for. I am still there today, but to be truthful, it is hard to show up to a place that you no longer respect. I don't let this affect me and how I do my job though. Being a pharmacy technician, I know I am helping patients. And I can now relate to some of the ones that we provide medication to. The clinic that I work at is a specialty clinic, so there are twelve floors of services that are provided. The twelfth floor specifically is the oncology floor. We don't treat children, it's only adults. But at times, it's still hard. During Lucas's treatment, I still showed up to work when I could. When I did, it was hard because I was still around the atmosphere of always talking about cancer. We dispensed the medications and helped oncology patients. I honestly, at times, don't know how I managed.

I can still clearly remember the first day that I had gone back to work after Lucas was diagnosed. The only person that I had informed of what was going on was my boss, and that was because I had to. She was courteous enough to ask me if I wanted her to inform my coworkers about what was going on because they kept asking her why I was gone. At this point, I had nicely declined and told her that I wasn't ready to let anybody know yet. She said that she understood and that if I needed anything to just let her know.

I walked in, and I felt that I was bombarded by my coworkers. I have great relationships with them, and so of course they were just trying to be concerned and make sure everything was okay. The only response that I gave before I walked out of the pharmacy crying so I could gain my composure back was that I didn't want to talk about it. I think I had gotten asked by about five different people, and thankfully, as I was making my way right back out, one of my coworkers who I call my work wife bluntly said, "Didn't you hear her? She doesn't want to talk about it. Leave her alone." That day felt very long, but I made it through. I think the only people that I had talked to were the patients, and that was because it's required for my job.

It took a while for me to get back into a groove and be okay being at work. I also became good at hiding my feelings. At the time, I didn't know it, but it would not be a good thing. Holding in emotions and feelings eventually catches up with you. Every day I went in, I still didn't talk much. Over time I was able to talk to different coworkers about what was going on. It was easier to talk about with some versus others. And each time I talked to someone new about it, I would start to cry. It got better over time. There were times when I needed to take a moment. But for the most part, I held my composure.

Working in the pharmacy did give me an advantage when it came to the medications Lucas would be taking. Because I had been familiar with them for the past five years, I already knew about them—what they were, what they were used for, and for the most part most of the side effects. It was also nice to have the pharmacists there, because when I did have questions, I was always bothering them to get answers.

Chapter 7

ADVENTURES

DURING THIS TIME, OUR FAMILY was very fortunate, and we were able to experience some amazing adventures. Our social worker had recommended Lucas for a wish through the Make-A-Wish Foundation. Since he was only four at the time of the wish, and he likes Disney, we decided to go to Disney World in Florida. This would also provide a great experience for my daughter. I didn't know that for this specific trip, Make-A-Wish has many connections. It was incredible to go on a trip and only have to worry about clothes and, most importantly, all of Lucas's medications and various things he would need. Everything was covered from flights to even spending money at the parks.

Our visit was booked for a weeklong stay. We were placed at a place called Give Kids the World. It is a village that is placed across eighty-four acres and is provided to families for a weeklong stay who have children with a critical illness. This place was truly magical, and even a week at this place didn't seem long enough to enjoy all of their festivities. Each family is given their own "house" to stay in. It's like a one-level duplex attached to another unit. It has two bedrooms, two bathrooms, a living room, a kitchen, and a dining room. The bathroom connected to the kids' room was huge with an enormous tub that they could take baths in. It even had a driveway! When you get there, they welcome you with a sign out front with your family's name on it.

The village consisted of multiple buildings and facilities that included the cafeteria, the castle, horse stables, a swimming pool and beach area, a salon to get your nails painted, many, many other buildings, and, most importantly, an ice-cream parlor. This was the most important building for the kids as they serviced ice all day, every day! It was open 24-7.

Each day of the week was designated to a specific event that would occur at the village. I don't recall which each day was for, but I do remember that Tuesday was for a pool party, and every Wednesday was a birthday party to celebrate the mayor's birthday. Yes, the village even has its own mayor, a rabbit. If you would like them to, one night you are there, the mayor and his wife will even come and tuck the children into bed and read them a bedtime story!

The castle was a special place. Each Make-A-Wish child got to create a special star that was numbered and placed on the wall of the castle tower. There were so many stars that covered the ceiling and tower that they are numbered and put into different areas that you are given the information, so when you go back to visit, you know where exactly to locate your star!

While we stayed here, we visited, of course, Disney World. This was an amazing experience. Not only did we get to visit all of the parks, but we were given a certain "genie" pass that gave us VIP advantages. We were able to skip the lines for all the adventures, including the lines for the fast pass that is offered. They truly make kids feel special and important. Emie and Lucas got to meet many characters throughout the parks. They collected many autographs in their special autograph books. The most important characters they met were Mickey and Minnie Mouse. There were so many details and places that I believe that it would be a book in itself to talk about. We visited Disney World for three days.

We also got to explore Sea World. This was a very cool experience as we got to see the last of the whale shows before they stopped performing. We got to see the whales along with many dolphin shows. Throughout the park were many rides and animal experiences. Besides the whales, the next best exhibit and ride was seeing the penguins. It was a very cold adventure, but it was well worth it!

We spent one day at Universal Studios, the Crayola exhibit, and did some sightseeing for a few days. One day we hung out in the village just playing in the pool. Universal Studios was another one of the places that were cool to experience. Being a Harry Potter fan, it was quite the experience to ride the train to Harry Potter Park. The rides in this area were amazing and unlike any of the rides you get at the basic amusement parks in Colorado.

It was such a nice adventure and something the kids still talk about. The week went by fast but felt long. And by the end of it, it was nice to finally be coming home. The two-hour time difference was rough. And by the end of it, I think our bodies were finally ready to be at home as well. It was hard to leave seventy-degree weather and come home to snow and twenty-degree weather!

We even were treated to luxury car services. We had a vehicle with a driver that picked us up from our house and took us to the airport. On the way home, we got to ride home in a limo!

Even after our Make-A-Wish trip, Lucas was still a part of their family. For the three years he went through chemotherapy, he was invited to an event that is hosted at the hospital each year. He got to go Christmas shopping and visit Santa to tell him what he wanted for Christmas. Each of these years, he was given Christmas dollars that he could use to shop for whom he wanted. He usually shopped for his cousins! He was taken into a room where there were tables full of presents. For each gift that he chose, he had to pay for it with one of his dollars. At the end of his shopping, there were Santa's elves to wrap and tag his presents for him!

The last event that he did with Make-A-Wish was their Fantasy Flight that they host with United Way. This was a unique experience as our family took a flight to the North Pole to meet Santa Clause himself! We went to DIA airport through security and hopped an hour flight to the North Pole! On our flight, the kids were given a Happy Meal so they could have a snack! Once we got to the North Pole, aka the hanger of United Way, we were given a tour. This included lunch and a bunch of goodies like cookies and desserts, some games to play, and of course—best of all—meeting Santa Claus and Mrs. Claus.

While we visited Santa in his special room, both Emie and Lucas were given many presents. They went home with so many new clothes and toys, it was mind-blowing! Emie is old enough that she knew it wasn't the North Pole, especially since once we left, our car was in the same parking lot we took a shuttle from to get to the airport! She is a good sport though and helped make sure that Lucas didn't catch on.

Chapter 8

EMIE

EMIE WAS ONLY SIX YEARS old and about halfway through first grade when all of this happened. It took me a while to realize the impact that this had on her as well. And at the very beginning of Lucas's diagnosis, she not only dealt with a lot herself but often at times felt like she was put on the back burner. Thankfully, she also had great individuals that helped take great care of her. Her first-grade teacher was helpful in more ways than I could have imagined. I had learned that her teacher's mom had died of leukemia, so she completely understood everything our family was dealing with. This felt like it was such a heavy burden taken off of my shoulders as I didn't have to explain anything to her about our situation. Spending the days with Emie, she could tell the toll it was taking on her. She was worried about Lucas and not sure exactly the extent of his condition. Emie is such a smart girl and has been very observant from a young age. Therefore she knew that Lucas was very sick. Emie's teacher noticed this and first off had Emie bring a picture of her and Lucas to school to put on her desk so she would always have him with her! She was also able to take a small toy of his to have at school so she could have something of his close to her. The next thing that she did was ask me if we could set up a "tutoring session" every Wednesday after school for thirty minutes. At first I thought that maybe Emie was starting to fall behind as her concerns were elsewhere. But the purpose of their sessions was so she could just hang out with Emie and give her one-on-one time so she felt special. They would read, play games, have snacks, and enjoy candy together.

She did this with Emie for about three months until the school year ended. To this day, she and Emie still keep in touch via email, and she still checks in on Emie since she moved school districts a few years later.

Another thing that her first-grade teacher did for Emie was to have the school purchase and donate tickets to our family for Disney on Ice for December 2015. This was amazing, and the kids had such a blast. I also didn't know that the school does other programs for families who are struggling. To our surprise, on top of this, the school donated Christmas gifts to both kids so they could enjoy presents from other students. I mean, she always went above and beyond. She gave Emie confidence and made sure she never felt left out nor worried.

We were once again very fortunate when Emie went into second grade. She was nervous about going to school and having a new teacher, but I guess there's always a blessing in disguise, and things happen for a reason. When we went to go meet her teacher before school started for the first time, she was nervous. But they both hit it off very well. And once again, we learned we had a teacher that knew exactly what we were going through. After explaining to her about Lucas and how Emie has been struggling, she was shocked. We both had encountered the same experiences to an extent. We learned that her teacher was also a cancer survivor of leukemia. This was her first-year teaching because she had finished chemotherapy about a year previously. She had gone through chemotherapy herself to battle cancer, so she knew everything that was involved. It's always nice to not have to talk about the situation, especially to someone new. It always seemed every time I would talk to someone new about what was going on, I would get very emotional and start crying. She helped Emie out a lot throughout the school year and always made sure to check on her to ensure she was doing well.

When you're thrown into something like this, you just seem to go with the flow. I felt that so many things were always coming up, and we were at the hospital a lot, so I didn't realize the toll this was taking on Emie. This was until one day she looked at me, crying, and said, "You don't love me anymore." This was a huge smack to the face and so devastating I felt like my heart had broken into a million pieces all over again. It also made me feel like I was a crappy parent and failing my daughter as a mom. It put into perspective why at certain times she would act out and try to mimic Lucas and his tantrums. Although this wasn't intentional because a lot of my time was with Lucas, it was still a reality check. Knowing that she felt unloved and unwanted made me check my perspective. It made me finally stop and think of everything that we were going through and that I needed to make time for her as well.

I was able to finally stop and rethink my actions and ensure that I was providing attention to her as well. She is such an amazing person and a daughter. She is an even more wonderful sister. She always made sure Lucas was comfortable and well taken care of. To this day, she still does. I truly couldn't have asked for a better daughter. I have made sure that I take the time to enjoy her and spend time together. We call them mommy and daughter days. I have also found foundations for her to be a part of so she can relate to other siblings and feel special herself outside of our family. She made a friend whose brother went through cancer, and she now has someone her age who she can relate to and share her feelings about certain things.

Years later, during one of Lucas's hospital stays, was when I truly realized how she must have felt. This was I believe about a year after the movie *Wonder* had come out. We were watching this movie for the first time, and when it got to the daughter's perspective of how her life was and how she felt at times when dealing with her brother's medical issues, I couldn't help but stop and think if this was in some way exactly how Emie felt at times. So many thoughts started running through my head at this point that I bawled like a baby. I think I cried for about twenty minutes, and Lucas even looked at me at one point and asked me why I was crying!

I felt for a while that I had failed Emie. Here I was, given this amazing gift of a child—smart, beautiful, caring, and so many other things that are beyond words that I needed to make sure that I was truly seeing her. I ended up just talking to her. From this point forward, we were able to just talk about our feelings, which we were never good at. This made our bond more special and her to realize that she could always come to me and let me know when she needed something if I wasn't always there. She will probably get mad at me for this, but she is my Toots and always will be!

It's strange, after truly taking the time to get to know Emie, I can't believe how incredible she is. I feel for her age; her maturity is much older. I can't believe that I took her for granted at one point in time. I have learned that time is something that we cannot get back, so we need to cherish every moment of it. I have learned to put my children first in a different way than I had originally thought as a parent. I have also made it my mission to take time off. No matter how many random days from work it needs to be, take time off. Just have a day as a reminder that I am blessed with grateful children. This time is the time that I have created so I can make sure that I am seeing my children and that I am spending time with them that they deserve.

Chapter 9

LUCAS

I DON'T EVEN KNOW WHERE to start this chapter. Wow, being three years old and having to go through everything that he did makes Lucas such an incredible boy, and I didn't know how strong he was until he went through this. There were even times that I would look at him for strength and inspiration to get through my struggles. There was so much that he had to endure over this time, there were times that I wasn't sure how he got through it all.

I've already described previously a lot of the details of things that he had to go through to become cancer-free. He is a strong, resilient kid. He never asked why this was happening to him or complained much about everything he had to go through. Heck, I can say he handle these three years of his life better than I would have as an adult!

One of the good moments I do recall is how Lucas made it through his journey. The first week that Lucas was diagnosed, we got our first visit from a volunteer. He had knocked on our door and asked if Lucas would like a blanket. I can't remember where they were donated from, but Lucas wanted one, so we got one for him. It was a smaller blanket that was blue and had yellow stars all over it. He clung to this blanket, and it got him through his journey. He was also fascinated with tags. And since this blanket had a tag, it made it that much better. Like I said before, he was a thumb-sucker. So whenever Lucas was having a difficult time, he had his blanket and his thumb! I have to admit, this did make things that much easier. It allowed him to sleep anywhere and everywhere with care in the world. Through all the hospital stays, he managed to sleep like a champ. He was not bothered by beeping machines, noise, light, etc.

He was given a special taggie lion by his cousins. This went everywhere with him, which gave him a sense of calmness as well. This lion had certain tags that were around his whole head. Of all the things Lucas was given over the years, these were by far his favorites. He was very sad when he dropped taggie somewhere, and he was lost. Many gracious people gave him another, but it was not the same. He has collected many stuffed animals over the three years, and he still has all of these animals as they are very special to him.

During his first in-clinic visit, he was also given a backpack from an organization called Bags of Fun. This backpack was filled with DVDs, books, a personal DVD player, some building blocks, and a cape with a mask. This cape and mask were his costumes. He wore this a lot, and it made him feel invincible!

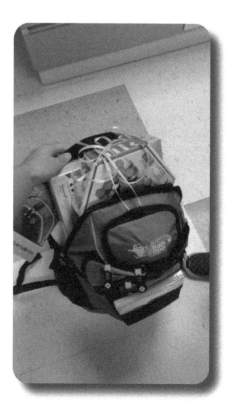

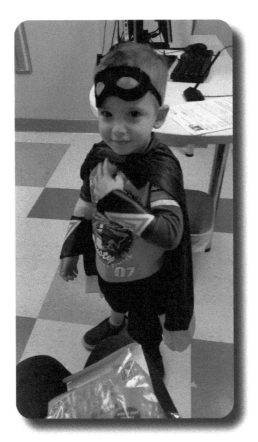

You don't know the treasures you have until they can be taken away. Throughout these three years, I learned a lot about Lucas. I can say that he is a survivor. I am very grateful for this as we did experience a time in his life that things could have gone differently. I know that not all families are blessed with this outcome, but I truly am. My handsome little man has grown and shown that he can overcome anything in life.

I think that this life experience has made him a gentle and loving person. It has taught us all a lot. Lucas is a shy boy, which I think from being secluded to hospital rooms a lot or being isolated due to risk of infections makes sense. He finds it hard to socialize and at times make new friends. The side effects of chemotherapy never really seem to be over. Yes, he is a cancer survivor. But you don't realize all the shit he has gone through and how it will affect him in the future until it is here.

Some things make him anxious and weary. He does not like big groups of people. Germs still worry him, not as much, but they do. He seems to finally have gotten over the shyness of his scar from where his port was. When he had his port, he would always make sure to wear a swim shirt when swimming. Now he sports it and knows that he is a strong person and will tell others that it's his scar from overcoming cancer. I've never thought of it, and I feel bad for never realizing it, but he has PTSD. He gets frightened when certain things are brought up or if he has to go somewhere that reminds him of what he has gone through.

There were many times I thought it was good that he got diagnosed so young and that he won't remember a lot of what happened. I guess this was partly wishful thinking. So many things have come up that should have been common sense, but they are things that I guess I never really thought about. Trying to find our new normal and live life after cancer is still an adventure in itself. There are some worries of new health factors: Will cancer come back? And how does Lucas truly deal with things?

One thing that has been constant for him is me. Anthony tends to tell me that I'm his safe place. I think this is because of all the time we've spent together and all the shit we've faced together. You can even consider us "cuddle buddies." We had spent so many nights in a hospital room snuggling together, making sure he always got sleep. He knows that no matter what, I will always be there for him. We do have an incredibly strong mother-son bond. For that, I am very thankful! I've gotten to know him in a way I may not have gotten to if things had been different. I've gotten to see his true strength and personality and see what kind of person he is. Cancer sucks! But I have to admit, I wouldn't change it because it led me to where we are and my wonderful, beautiful children.

Chapter 10

SELF-REFLECTION

THIS JOURNEY WAS LIFE-ALTERING. I learned so much about myself and others that I look at life in a whole new light now. I went from being depressed to being angry to being thankful among many other feelings that I didn't know you could have. Not only did this affect me, but it also affected my marriage, my relationship with my kids, and my relationships with family and friends. I became resentful toward some people, lost respect for others, and found those that I could depend on when I needed them most.

I don't think my brain ever fully comprehended everything this would entail for our family to go through. It felt like it was a whirlwind, and I never could catch up. To this day, there are times where I think back and don't fully understand things still and think, *Did we go through all of this?*

First off, this was not easy on my marriage. At times, I even felt angry at Anthony and myself for that matter. He was always good at hiding any kind of emotions, and at times I felt it was hard to talk to him about certain things as he didn't like to talk about them. It made things hard, especially when a lot of the times the responses that I did get were "I don't know, but things will be all right." Anthony is a private person, so I'm not going to go into a whole lot of detail here about some of the struggles our marriage entailed. I will say this, though: he is by far a great dad.

There were times where I struggled more than others, and I feel this was because I was a MOM. I took Lucas to 99 percent of his appointments. I gave him his medications; I was the one that would be up with him when he wasn't feeling well. I stayed with him during his hospital visits. I endured the brunt of everything. And it takes a toll no matter how strong you are. This could partly do with the way that I am built. I tend to think that my way is always the right way, and that things should be done exactly the way I want. I tended to take everything on by myself to make sure that things were done my way and to my standards. Looking back, maybe this was so I could make sure that I was not missing anything when it came to Lucas and his treatment. There were even times where I felt I didn't have enough strength to get through this, but then I would look at Lucas and tell myself to suck it up. He was the one that was going through the hard part, I was just there to ensure he got everything he needed to become cancer-free. Kids truly are resilient, and he was a strong fighter.

At the time, I didn't realize it, but work was also a constant reminder of cancer. As I mentioned earlier, I work at a specialty clinic. The pharmacy is located on the first floor, and of course we dispense prescriptions to patients from their visits. The twelfth floor is the oncology floor. I think they put oncology at the top because the view is amazing, and patients can reel in the view of Downtown Denver while they are getting their infusions. Anyways, it never really dawned on me. But every day that I would show up to work, I was always around cancer patients and talk about chemo medications, treatments, and patients and their journeys. I never had an outlet or a place to go that I didn't have to think about cancer. At times it was hard, and on bad days that I had to deal with tough patients, I found myself taking breaks and going down the hall just to cry. I didn't want to, and I would try hard to fight back the tears. But once they started to fall, there was no stopping.

Even though work was a constant reminder, not all was bad. As I talked about before, people try to empathize with you and try to understand what you're going through. But no matter how hard they try, it just isn't meaningful. I'm not trying to be rude, but until you have faced it, you can't fully endure all the pain and thoughts that go through one's mind. Because of my journey with Lucas, I was able to see our chemotherapy patients and their families in a whole new light.

I was able to connect with them on a whole new level and understand all the fears, anxiety, and different types of emotions that they were going through. At times it made me enjoy my job a little more, and at times I struggled. I learned how to have a conversation that met their needs. Trust me, there are many different discussions one could have about certain things. You could talk about their day, if they were just diagnosed, if they were far along within treatment, if cancer came back, how they were coping amongst many other topics. I also learned how to have conversations with family members. Most of the time, they are scared. But it's nice to be able to relate and remind them to be kind to themselves and to make sure that they are taking care of themselves as well. Because like I learned, often enough you put yourself on the back burner and tend to forget about yourself.

When Lucas was hospitalized for the long haul, I didn't know how to cope, and I didn't like to talk about everything that was going on. I didn't even like to talk about my feelings with Anthony. One reality that sunk in was when I was having a conversation with our social worker. During our conversation, she asked me if I had been able to say the C word. I was so confused, and so many words came to mind that I didn't know where she was going with this. I think she could tell I had no clue what she was talking about because she finally said, "You know, the C word, *cancer.*" I realized that I had not said it. I never acknowledge it, and it took me probably a good four to six months to use the word *cancer* when telling people what was wrong with Lucas. To this day, I feel I still struggle about certain topics. But throughout all of this, I did learn a lot about myself, how tough I was, and I managed to find my voice.

After a recommendation from a coworker about an antidepressant and being informed that there's nothing to be ashamed of about being on one for help with all the shit I was going through, I talked to my doctor. I did get on medication, and I started to see a therapist. To this day, if needed, I still talk to my therapist. I learned that therapy is a great outlet and that you can be open and honest with a person who won't judge you. Don't get me wrong, this took me a long time to realize and to be able to open up and talk about certain aspects of my life that I had always kept to myself. Of course, because of society and how judgmental my parents could be, I kept this to myself for quite a while. I don't think I dared to open up to them about it until after Lucas was done with all of his treatment. To this day, they still don't understand, especially my mom. So at times it is still hard. However, because I was helping myself, I did what I thought was best for me. After a while, I found myself not caring. I had been through some traumatic shit in my life, and I'm sure others have as well. I started opening up and talking about it, and I felt good about it. Either people could relate and be too ashamed to talk about it as well, or people didn't respond. I realized I'm my person. You can take me as I am and accept it, or you can keep walking! I think, as adults, we finally get to a point in life where we're just so tired of being judged and trying to live up to the standards of society. We are all entitled to ourselves, our beliefs, and our opinions. You may not like it but, at least, try to respect it. Everyone has different perspectives, that's what makes us our own person and also what makes us human.

At one point, one of the ways that I tended to cope with everything and feel "numb" was to drink. Now I'm not saying that I would get trashed and be drunk. Although I do have to admit, there may have been a couple of times where I did this on a weekend. Don't get me wrong though, that was the thought in my head. I turned to wine. I don't know why wine. Maybe in the back of my head, I convinced myself that this was the healthiest choice of alcohol. But wine it was. Now you may not believe me, but I did at least limit myself. I would not drink more than two glasses of wine, but I was drinking two glasses of wine every night for a while. On a really bad day, it would be three glasses just so I could feel a tad bit of a greater buzz to try and ease the pain of all the things around me. In the back of my head, I knew that I shouldn't abuse alcohol like this and that could be one of the reasons that I wouldn't allow myself to drink more. Also after two glasses of wine, I would be feeling a good buzz anyways because of the antidepressant that I was on. I know, I know, I should know better than to drink on an antidepressant. I mean, there is a warning label on the bottle itself. But I also work in a pharmacy, so I should know better. I think that if I knew I drank more than two as well, I couldn't provide the care for my kids that they had deserved. There are also the thoughts of shame that come into your mind as well. Growing up, you're taught about different aspects and how you should behave. Being an "alcoholic" is not acceptable, and I didn't want to feel ashamed or like I was letting my family down. All of these combined, I think, played a huge factor. I'm the type of person who always tends to do what is right so I can please others and not let anybody down. It sucks. For just once I wish I could be whoever I want to be and not have a freakin' worry in the world. But in this case, it was probably for the best. In retrospect, I can see how people drink to escape reality and the things that they are going through in life.

I don't recall how long that I did this for, but it must have been for some time. After some time, Anthony confronted me and told me that I needed to get my act together. A reality check is what it was, and it made me reevaluate what I was doing and how I was truly coping with everything and all my feelings. It made me realize that I wasn't doing it very well. I tried to keep myself occupied as best as I could. And thinking back, this could be why my brain never caught up and recognized all the reality of everything. I put myself in a box and bottled everything up, which is not a healthy way to cope.

During Lucas's treatment, I ended up getting some tattoos. They are meaningful and pertain to both of my children. I knew that I always wanted some but never could decide on what I wanted to get. While I was going through this, I learned a lot not only about myself but also about many different things in life. My favorite flowers are orchids, and the meaning behind this flower is love. Easy enough, I would get an orchid for each of my children to represent them and the love that I have for them. Each also has its initials along with them and attached to Lucas's in a golden ribbon to represent childhood cancer. It's interesting though, tattoos are painful, I guess, depending on where you get them. I already had two, both of my kid's footprints that I stamped when they were only seven months old. These are on each of my feet. Painful, a little bit, but at the time to me, it wasn't too bad because I compared it to the labor pains I endured when I was giving birth to Emie. I know, this might seem odd. But compared to trying to give birth without an epidural is some serious pain! So these weren't so bad. For the orchid tattoos, I decided to get them placed on both of the insides of my biceps. Again, this spot can be tender and painful. I'm not gonna say that it wasn't painful in certain spots, but again, I compared it to other pain. During this time, this was when Lucas was first diagnosed. After watching what he was going through, I just told myself that I wasn't allowed to feel any pain because this pain was minor compared to everything that he was going through. Again, the word "numb" comes to mind. During Lucas's treatment, I got a total of three tattoos. The two for Emie and Lucas, and the third was for me. It was a mental reminder of how I need to treat myself as well as others. It's a phrase on the inside of my right forearm that says "stay humble, work hard, be kind." It also has a small yellow daffodil to represent March, my birth month flower. It's interesting to reflect and see how your emotions are triggered by pain and how you can feel numbness when there is darkness in your life.

While we were receiving help from nonprofit organizations, it was such a relief to know that there are people out that, specifically for families with children battling cancer, willing to help. This had meant a lot to me, and I was and still am very grateful for all of those who helped us out. It also reminded me of when I was younger and would volunteer and the great feeling that I had, knowing that I was helping others when they needed it the most. This led me to realize that although through my job as a pharmacy technician and while I was helping patients that I truly was not happy doing what I was doing. I wanted to do something else. So on impulse, I enrolled in school. While Lucas was going through chemotherapy, I did online school so I could still work as well. It took me almost two years, but I got my master's in nonprofit management. My goal is to open up my nonprofit organization so I could help other families that were through or had gone through what my family has gone through. It has taken a lot of hard work and dedication, but my organization has been founded, The Lumies Foundation, a mash-up of both Emie and Lucas. Go figure, when they were fighting one day, and I was trying to get both of their attention. Lumies came out, and that's how the name was born!

This was not easy, but I managed. I managed with the help of Anthony at times taking the kids on weekends out of the house so

I could write my ten to twelve-page papers that were due for certain
assignments for various courses that I took. I would also use my lunch
breaks to get work done. A lot of my evenings after the kid's home-
work was done, I would get back on and make sure I was making my
deadlines for assignments. Through this, I learned a lot about charity
work and all the different types of help that are out there even beyond
pediatric cancer.

At times I felt so insecure and unsure about myself and who I
was. I also wasn't sure who I was meant to be. These doubts haunt
you and sometimes can overtake you. It took a lot for me to come
out of my shell and finally realize that I am my person. I am who I
want to be, regardless of what others think. If they don't like it, then
that's not on me, that's on them, and they can deal with it, not me! I
realized that I was always trying to be perfect or be someone else just
so I would be liked or feel good about myself. It took me a long time,
but I finally realized that nobody is perfect. I feel that perfection is
hype. No matter how hard you try, you will never be perfect because
there is always another problem or issue that you will face in life. I
feel that I am still a work in progress, but I am learning how to have
faith in myself.

In the first sessions of my therapy, I don't think I talked much at
all, and I remember sitting on the couch in my therapist's office and
looking around thinking, How did I get here? Aren't the fucked-up
people the ones that should be here? Not that I'm not fucked up in
my ways since all of this, but it's one of those reality checks that life
is not perfect. I think it took me a full year to fully open up and start
being truthful with my therapist about all the shit I was going through
and how I truly felt. I learned so much about myself and established
things from my past that I forgot that I was good at, that it was a good
self-reflection. It taught me that I needed to remember to take care of
myself and do things for myself. That way I could continue to take care
of my family.

Through therapy and many different trials of antidepressants, I
can say that I finally found myself again. I still struggle with self-con-
fidence at times and hate when I'm indecisive about things and can't
decide on what I feel is best. I often feel like a blank canvas, and I'm

not sure where to start. I guess that's why I'm still a work in progress. I'm still trying to work on myself and find who I am. I do know that I am a strong and determined person who will go far. Let's start there!

Strength in Numbers

LISTED BELOW SHOWS WHAT LUCAS went through during his three years of chemotherapy.

IV chemo: 64 doses

Oral chemo: 1,063 days

Oral steroids (chemo only): 207 days (If we went by dose, it would be 414.)

Subcutaneous chemo: 8 doses

Spinal taps: 22

Red blood cell transfusions: 3

Platelet transfusions: 6

Hospital admissions: 5

Clinic visits: 73 (This number includes clinic visits for spinal taps.)

Emergency Department visits during treatment: 14

During his chemotherapy, Lucas also received Beads of Courage. This was a way we could keep track and show his courage of what he was going through. There are twenty-nine different beads. Lucas did not receive all twenty-nine, but he did receive quite a bit. His collection consisted of beige (bone marrow aspirate), white (chemotherapy/immunizations), blue (clinic visit/infusion/medication log), magenta (ER/unusual occurrence/ambulance), brown-and-face bead (hair loss), purple (infusions), yellow (inpatient admission), lime (isolation/fever/neutropenia), orange (line place for port), tortoise (lumbar puncture), bumpy (medication challenges—learning/taking), black (pokes—IV starts, blood draws, injections, port access), star (surgery), light green (test/scans), red (transfusions), rainbow (care team visit—PT). There are also milestone beads that he received as well—special selection (special accomplishments/recognition), glass selection (an act of courage), and purpleheart (completion of treatment).

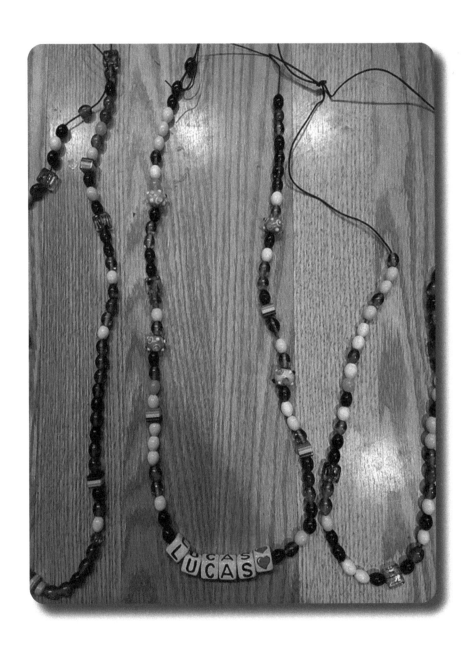

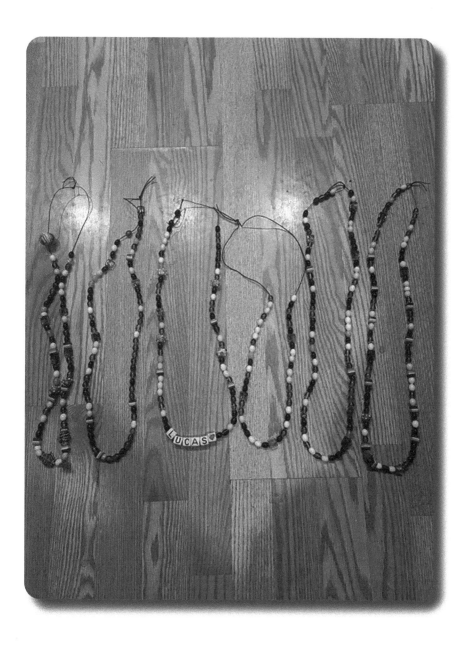

About the Author

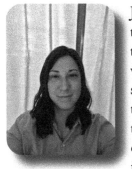

JENIFER HIGGINS IS A MARRIED mother of two, business owner, grant writer, and pharmacy technician. She is a Colorado native. She began working at the early age of fourteen, serving senior citizens at an assisted living center. At sixteen, she purchased her first car, even learning to change the oil and tires! She has always been driven, allowing her to receive a bachelor's degree in biology and a master's in nonprofit management. In 2015, her son was diagnosed with acute lymphoblastic leukemia, turning her world upside down. She has always loved to write but rediscovered writing as an outlet to cope with her three-year journey of ups and downs during this difficult time. Jenifer enjoys kickboxing, running, writing, arts and crafts, and, most of all, spending time with her loved ones.

CPSIA information can be obtained
at www.ICGtesting.com
Printed in the USA
LVHW052011200422
716062LV00010B/66